Clinical Futures

D1080571

Clinical Futures

Edited by

MARSHALL MARINKER
Visiting Professor of General Practice, GKT, University of London, UK

MICHAEL PECKHAM
Director, School of Public Policy, University College London, UK

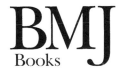

© BMJ Books 1998
BMJ Books is an imprint of the BMJ Publishing Group

All rights reserved. No part of this publication may be reproduced, stored in a retrieval system, or transmitted, in any form or by any means, electronic, mechanical, photocopying, recording and/or otherwise, without the prior written permission of the publishers.

First published in 1998
by BMJ Books, BMA House, Tavistock Square,
London WC1H 9JR

British Library Cataloguing in Publication Data

A catalogue record for this book is available from the British Library

ISBN 0-7279-1231-3

Typeset by Apek Typesetters, Nailsea, Bristol
Printed and bound by Latimer Trend, Plymouth.

Contents

Contributors

John Bell
Nuffield Professor of Clinical Medicine, University of Oxford, UK

David Delpy
Hamamatsu Professor of Medical Photonics, Department of Medical Physics and Bioengineering, University College London, UK

John Grimley Evans
Professor of Clinical Geratology, University of Oxford, UK

Leslie Iversen
Visiting Professor, Department of Pharmacology, University of Oxford, UK

Marshall Marinker
Visiting Professor of General Practice, GKT, University of London, UK

Catherine Peckham
Professor of Paediatric Medicine, Institute of Child Health, University of London, UK

Michael Peckham
Director, School of Public Policy, University College London, UK

Philip Poole-Wilson
Professor of Cardiology, National Heart and Lung Institute, Imperial College School of Medicine, London, UK

Karol Sikora
Chief, WHO Cancer Programme, International Agency for Research on Cancer, Lyon, France; Professor of International Cancer Medicine, Imperial College School of Medicine, London, UK

Foreword

This book is the third in a series initiated and supported by Merck Sharp and Dohme. The first two, *Controversies in Health Care Policies* (1994), and *Sense and Sensibility in Health Care* (1996), examined some of the paradoxes and dilemmas consequent on the attempt to provide an excellent health service in the public domain. The National Health Service, like so many other health services in the developed world, continues to struggle with policy imperatives that reflect rising public expectation, an ageing population, the fundamental principle of fairness, and the constraints of pre-determined and fixed resources.

Now, in *Clinical Futures*, the third book in this series, the editors Marshall Marinker and Michael Peckham have invited a number of the country's leading clinical researchers to examine another set of policy imperatives – those deriving from the possibilities of future medical advance. Their essays suggest that medical science and technology are about to transform our personal lives, our sense of identity, and the very structure of our social life. We are left with tantalising glimpses of unfamiliar health care scenarios, professional roles and tasks not yet invented, and unprecedented moral choices for the public.

It is a pleasure to welcome this innovative book on the occasion of the 50th anniversary of the National Health Service, as a contribution to that celebration, and to the hopes that we all invest in the next fifty years of its history.

Vincent Lawton
Managing Director
MSD Ltd (UK)
Vice President MSD (Europe) Inc

Preface

This book is not intended to be an exercise in clairvoyance but rather an attempt to examine some of the trends and discoveries that will shape the future of clinical practice over the coming decades. What emerges is a guide to the sorts of developments and consequences which it would be unwise to interpret as firm predictions but foolish to dismiss as fantasy. These essays should be read as a reconnaissance across the boundary of present and future, and therefore across the boundary of what is known and what might be known.

Since the content of the book was to be future orientated, we thought to compose it on the Internet. Each author was invited to nominate up to five discussants from similar or adjacent scientific disciplines. Discussants were asked to comment on and contribute to drafts of chapters as they were posted on to a *Clinical Futures* web-site set up for us by our publishers, BMJ Books. The aim was to stimulate a fresh, interactive approach with diverse inputs shaping and modelling the final product.

Although our authors were writing for a non-specialist readership, inevitably some of the terms that some employ will be unfamiliar. To avoid completely the jargon of current biotechnology would have placed too great a burden on the specialist writers. They would have been forced to create dense thickets of parenthetical explanations in the text, in which the reader could easily be lost. The editors have taken the view that the lay reader may safely surf the occasional arcane passages, without losing the broad thrust of the arguments being adduced, or the broad picture that is being painted. We rejected the solution of a glossary on the grounds that its use would unhelpfully impede the reader.

We have many people to thank: our authors for their enthusiasm for the project and their adherence to tight deadlines; the chapter discussants for their invaluable input and forbearance in coping with the teething problems of the Internet technology; BMJ Publishing Group, and in particular Mary Banks and Alex Stibbe for their support, and Tony Delamothe who encouraged us to keep the web-site technology going.

MSD Limited have given generous and unconditional financial and moral support to this project from its inception, and we particularly want to record our thanks to Kate Tillett, MSD Director of External Affairs, for her personal enthusiasm and commitment. Richard Smith, Editor, *BMJ*, was the other invaluable support whose advice and encouragement were so helpful.

Sally Welham acted throughout as a troubleshooter, providing coherence and constant support to the two editors: our debt to her tact, skills and input is immense. Finally we would like to place on record the fun we had in working with each other on this unusual project which we see as the start of a process, not an end in itself. We hope that this sense of enjoyment and adventure will be conveyed to the reader in the essays that follow.

Marshall Marinker and Michael Peckham

1   Looking and leaping

Marshall Marinker

> Time will say nothing but I told you so,
> Time only knows the price we have to pay;
> If I could tell you I would let you know.

WH Auden. Collected Shorter Poems, 1966

There is a burgeoning literature on the future of health-care policy, much of it stemming from the perspectives of political and social theorists, economists and managers. These perspectives have, for many decades, dominated thinking about the conduct and future of the NHS. Their speculations have had to take account of such powerful forces as political will, economic performance, and social, demographic and morbidity trends.

This book was designed to offer a view of the future of medicine, health services and policy, from the perspectives of current clinical research. Seven areas of research were selected (genetics, engineering, brain function, cancer, heart and circulation, children's health, and ageing) in an attempt to provide a series of reconnaissances into the future of health, care, and society.

Time

The icon of our age is the exponential curve. Wherever we look – at Man's technological mastery over the past millennium, or at the rate of increase in computer power over the past decades, the long, long, almost horizontal line of crawling incremental progress suddenly erupts into this dizzy upward leap, climbing like a Saturn rocket almost vertically into the heavens. Something marvellous and unprecedented is happening to our sense of the future. We are leaping into it.

Leaders of Governments or Quangos or professional bodies tend to measure time in relatively short units determined by their "terms of office". This makes internal political sense, but serves uncer-

1

tainly the needs of national or institutional planning. Freeman Dyson, in his book *Imagined Worlds*,[1] suggests that the decade is the basic unit of historical time, which he describes as "the normal horizon of human activities" – the timescale for educating a child, preparing for a career, developing a current technology. The decade is the common temporal currency of most policy making. It is also the timespan of present research. The coming decade, says Dyson, will see the skies mapped by the new technology of Digital Astronomy, and Man mapped by the Human Genome Project.

He begins his look at the future with the span of 100 years (longer than the youngest reader is likely to survive). In that time he believes that we will have begun to colonise the Moon and possibly Mars, and learned better how to manage a sustainable life on Earth. He concludes his look at the future with a span of a million years. This extends back to the dawn of *Homo erectus*, and forward to a time when our species will have evolved into a new family of differentiated creatures occupying ecological niches far into the galaxy. By then, *Homo sapiens* may survive only as a protected species inhabiting the nature reserve of planet Earth.

Our choice of a 50-year purview was not entirely arbitrary – for example in the year in which we write the UK National Health Service is celebrating its fiftieth anniversary. On Dyson's analysis, 50 years offers some expectation of credible extrapolation and speculation. Even so, our writers found half a century a tad ambitious.

Habits of thought

Inevitably, our view of the future is shaped by the assumptions of the present: the poet Goethe suggested that Man only sees what he already knows. All the authors, leaders in their fields of research, are engaged in what Thomas Kuhn[2] called "normal science". That is to say they are pushing to the boundary of explanation and utility the concepts, models, vocabulary, the methods – what Thomas Kuhn called collectively the "paradigms" – of their fields.

Denkstil (a German term meaning "style of thought") pervades current scientific research, is powerful, productive but can also be misleading, because it shapes a world constructed on assumptions unchallenged by those small inconvenient elements of evidence that do not fit with current received wisdom. A recently quoted example concerns the teratogenic effect of thalidomide.[3] The effects of alcohol on the fetus had been known since Biblical days.

In 1941, it had been established that maternal rubella could damage a growing fetus. Yet an almost unchallenged assumption persisted among clinicians that the human placenta gave perfect protection to the fetus.

The medical historian Ann Dally suggests that such scientific assumptions can be unconsciously reinforced by social attitudes. She speculates that the nineteenth century (and subsequent) belief in the placenta as a perfect barrier against damaging influences in the environment might have been reinforced by the Victorian tendency to put "woman" on a pedestal. This, she believes, led to idealisation of the womb as well as of the woman. Although her views (about the predictability of the effects of thalidomide on the fetus) have been contested, she concludes that her analysis of the historical context of the thalidomide disaster suggests that there was more to the story of the thalidomide tragedy than the "out of the blue" theory suggests.

What must perforce be missing from our reconnaissances into the future is the unpredictable, the product of a clinical science which would result from fundamental challenges to present assumptions. Such a necessarily silent but parallel future is the uninvited ghost at this feast of our next 50 years of clinical progress. I am not forecasting that this ghost will actually materialise during the timespan of our story. Far from it. I doubt the imminent advent of a new revolutionary bioscience, because the current biological paradigms continue to yield such riches. The theories of special relativity and quantum physics, that date from the beginning of the twentieth century, provided such novel, fundamental and fruitful insights into the physical world, that they still dominate its exploration, and our imaginations. Similarly, in terms both of materially important and useable findings, and of funding and academic careers, biology remains in thrall to the explanations and explorations consequent on the description of DNA. That breakthrough dates back only to the mid years of the twentieth century. Such rare world-changing epiphanies as the DNA story cast a blinding light over the scientific imagination, so that little beyond what it illuminates can yet be discerned. But surprises will always surprise: "If I could tell you, I would let you know".

The scientist may be driven by what Sir Peter Medawar called "imaginative conjectures", but these do not arise unbidden from some dream-world. They are rooted in everything that has gone before. What has gone before inevitably influences where to look next, and what to recognise, but it cannot accommodate surprise.

3

At the turn of the last century, such was the volume of traffic that it was predicted that the streets of London would very shortly become impassable because of the depth of horse-droppings. Nor can the past reliably construct the timescale of prediction.

In 1970 Marvin Minsky[4] forecast that a computer with the (artificial) intelligence of the average human being would be available "in 3–8 years", with a machine at genius level very soon thereafter. Julius Comroe[5] in one of his essays about the value of hindsight in thinking about the future, warns of the dangers of false predictions, especially by eminent scientists: "Francis Bacon could not believe that the earth goes around the sun; Galileo could not accept Kepler's evidence that the planets move in ellipses . . .".

If the direction and success and timing of invention are so uncertain, what do these essays illuminate? I suggest three linked insights. First, how health scientists, currently engaged at the cutting edge of their disciplines, believe that they are shaping our futures as human organisms and as future societies. Second, their perceptions of the opportunities and hazards of this future so that we can begin to plan for (or perhaps in some events to plan against) what they portend. Third, a demonstration of what Jacob Bronowski[6] described as the three moral "givens" of the scientific mind: creativity, the habit of truth, and the sense of human dignity. To these I would add, on much of the evidence in the essays that follow, a tendency to optimism.

Demography

Two demographic trends are evident. First, more individuals than ever before are surviving into the sixth and later decades of life. Since most of the illnesses with which we are now faced stem from the genetic vulnerabilities and environmental challenges that declare themselves increasingly with age, the burden of ill health may well increase at the population level, while at the individual level it will probably substantially diminish.

Second, currently the level of childbirth does not achieve a replacement of the UK population. Since our NHS is funded from taxation, not from investment in insurance, the health-care burden of the retired old on the employed young may be judged unsustainable by the early decades of the next century.

As John Grimley Evans suggests, the solution to this paradox will come not from changing the cold facts of economics, but from changing our attitudes, from recognising certain social and psychological imperatives: "Far from being a social incubus, the new caste of older people freed from the tangling nets of employment and patronage, could be the grey guardians of all our freedoms."

In Chapter 7, an array of spectacular future interventions is described, aimed at the safe production of healthy newborns. Catherine Peckham predicts that things ". . . will change as society invests in childbearing as a means of assuring stability, prosperity, competitiveness and cultural vigour". In this there is the suggestion that technology will only provide the illusion of convenience and choice about if and when to have a baby, and that there will always be a strong and overriding Darwinian drive at work, to achieve survival as a critical social mass. Grimley Evans underscores the likely intensity of this procreative drive: "In a rational and compassionate world" he asks, "would anyone question the right of a woman of 60 having a baby or a widow to conceive a child from the sperm of her dead husband?"

In future more of us will survive longer, fitter than before, with a foreshortening of the time lapse between the onset of disability and death. Grimley Evans paints a dark picture of old age punctuated by the endless affliction of TV soap operas – euthanasia by *Neighbours*. He raises the question of the "medicalisation" of ageing. The alternative to such medicalisation may be that the many forms of immunological decline in old age will be declassified as disease. In this sense the term "disease" could in future be reserved for those conditions when there was an *intention to treat*.

Redefining disease

Since the eighteenth century, although the dominant metaphors changed with the changing fashions for structural or functional explanations of "cause" and "mechanism", diseases have been recognised by their *common* characteristics. The pictures that emerged were averages, composites of innumerable examples derived from *populations* of patients. Consequently the individual disease, the patients particular condition, only bore a general resemblance to this abstract template. This gap between clinical science and the particular patient's complaint was most noticeable in the countless encounters with "unselected" patients in British general practice – patients who presented their problems not as fully fledged diseases, but as still inchoate and unorganised illnesses.

Nothing so illuminates the limitations of these "solid" older concepts of disease as the advent of "evidence-based medicine".[7] This was an approach to clinical standard-setting that took the results from large research studies, aggregating the data from very many of them, and presenting them as guidelines, protocols, and clinical algorithms, which could assume the status of clinical instructions; instructions often resisted by clinicians. Far from reflecting a poor respect for science, this resistance may have reflected the doctor's instinctual understanding of the highly complex relationship between study findings, aggregated data, and clinical judgement.

In Chapter 2 John Bell explains that a lack of precision (at the genetic level) in diagnosis at the point of entry into trials results in a hidden heterogeneity in the study population, so that diverse subgroups are lumped together, rendering uncertain the application of the results to the individual patient. Genetic technology offers the prospect of quite a different and more profound level of diagnosis.

Of diagnosis, and therefore also of treatment. Since there is no such person as the average patient, there can be no average drugs for her disease, the sort of pharmaceutical approximations that today constitute the best available treatment. In future the technology of "pharmacogenomics" will make it possible to mix cocktails of drugs precisely to match the genetic characteristics of the patient's "receptors". Such a revolution in therapeutics will challenge the pharmaceutical industry to adjust from today's international mass-markets, to a diversity of clinical micro-markets.

The seemingly solid models of what is wrong with the patient, derived from past bio-engineering metaphors, are disaggregated in the solvent of these new insights from genomics and enhanced body imaging. The advent of such personalised diagnoses will result in a very different classification from the present one, expressing a deeper level of understanding transecting and redrawing the now familiar territorial boundaries of medical specialisms.

The public health

Perhaps the most profound change in our perception of disease will come from the inexorable quest to intervene earlier and earlier in the process of its natural history. Now, as this imperative is extended to scrutinising the genetic make-up of the healthy individual in order to predict future mischief, the boundary between being a person and being a patient quite disappears. Just as the nature of diagnosis and the specificity of treatment change in the light of genomics, so does the concept of risk. Philip Poole-Wilson in Chapter 6 questions the utility of the attempt to apply what is known about an increasingly large array of markers for heart disease (including elements of diet, behaviour, social position and perception) to statements about individual risk. These "risk factors" have strong predictive value for the health of populations, but weak predictive value for the health of individuals. The consequence has been the growth of a misdirected special-interest consumerism in health care, at the cost of a more productive public health agenda.

It seems that genetic research, far from ushering in a deterministic view of morbidity, will underscore the limitations of a nature/nurture dichotomy. Catherine Peckham writes that in 50 years' time the ". . . 'nature versus nurture' debate will then seem as crude and as sinister, to us, as turn-of-the-century eugenics concepts do today".

Many of the environmental risk factors touched on in this book (for example, the increased risk of heart disease among those whose work allows little latitude for choice and flexibility) reflect the social relationships that we have taken as "given" (for example, in the workplace), without sufficiently reflecting on the relationship between feelings and health. Research into the persistently higher rates of morbidity and mortality among the poorer members of society suggests that the causes of the differences between the classes go deeper than the deprivation of material goods: "The social consequences of people's differing circumstances in terms of stress, self-esteem and social relations may now be one of the most important influences on health".[8]

All this reinforces the view from public health (a crucial health discipline, but necessarily underrepresented in this book about clinical medicine) that the pursuit of better health will require much more than modifying our biological machinery. We will need public health thinking comparable in scope and radicalism with what is foreshadowed here in biotechnology. A politics shaped by the goals of health, would as a consequence have to discover new ways of reconciling the paradoxical goals of personal freedom and social justice. In political terms responsibility for health care would be relegated to a *Department of Illness*. The Government as a whole would then be obliged to accept the implication that in all its policy making (on housing, education, crime, social security, and so on), it must, in the fullest sense, assume the responsibilities of a *Department of Health.*

Staying human

Although the importance of the patient's constitution in determining the nature and course of disease has been recognised since the advent of Greek and Arabic medicine, the possibilities of genetic screening now open unfamiliar windows on our individual genealogy, the future history of our personal lives, and the constitutional bequests that we impose on future generations.

Increasingly the twenty-first century view of disease will move further away from the image of illness as affliction, to that of illness as biography. The term "biographical medicine" has until now been reserved for the patient's narrative – for the impact of illness on life, and of life on illness. Will illness now increasingly come to be seen by the patient not simply as a biological accident, a fault in the machine, an environmental assault, but rather as an expression of the essential self?

The present availability of tests for a variety of disorders like Huntington's disease and cystic fibrosis, and the potential of genetic testing eventually to reveal the "expressivity" of these genes, may reveal information about the date of onset and the severity. In many relatively common diseases (for example, cancer, cardiovascular disease, diabetes and Alzheimer's), it will be possible to construct elaborate genetic profiles of susceptibility.

What will we make of this new information? It is one thing for the patient today to learn that she is at risk – for example of a stroke because she has high blood pressure. This is, after all, not a specific prediction about her future. It is an observation based on the study of large groups of individuals, about the order of risks in groups of people similar to her in some medically relevant respects. The risk may be run by a majority, but an unspecifiable one, of the group to which she happens to belong, but by no means by all members of the group. There is nothing *personal* implied. It would be quite another thing for the patient to learn that she is personally programmed to develop a fatal disease, and to know approximately when – to know that this fact is written into the very fabric of her body. Thankfully Bell suggests that genetic prognosis may not be quite so dismally accurate. TS Eliot was right to comment that ". . .

human kind/ Cannot bear very much reality".

The power of genetic technology to diagnose will for the foreseeable future greatly outstrip its power to prevent or intervene. The underlying question is this: when the technology changes, can the ethics remain unchanged and absolute, or are they relative, contingent on what we can know and what we can do? When the tools are to hand with which to screen for major diseases, at what point will a genetic screening programme merge with a policy of eugenics, seductively presented in the guise of public health?

The last time that our species was materially moulded by natural selection, we were hunting and gathering on the savannah, and life for the majority was brutish and short. Having moved far beyond Darwinian natural selection, we seem poised to enter a new era of iatric selection. And this culling of the "bad genes" will not be without its biological hazards. Many of the genes that now make us prey to diseases in later life, convey benefit earlier in life, or at an earlier stage in our evolution.[9] As Bell suggests, the elimination of "bad" genes may not have unmixed "good" consequences. Whether or not we will view future iatric selection as "unnatural" or "undesirable" will depend on our deepest instincts about what it means to be human. If science and technology pose these uncomfortable questions, can the clinical scientists help to answer them?

We may be at one of those defining moments in the development of species, when things take a sudden turn, akin to whatever global environmental upheaval resulted in the disappearance of the dinosaurs. If so, the driving force for this change will not explode from the cosmos, but from within our own human brains. As *Homo sapiens* prepares to depart, *Designer Man* may already have made her tentative appearances within the half-century ahead.

Configurations

How will the new clinical technologies influence the structures and functions of the future NHS? In Chapter 3 David Delpy describes the coming developments in biometric sensors, tele-medicine, robotics, and unimaginable machine–body interfaces. Such innovation must force a massive reinvention of health services and organisations. These have scarcely changed in the UK over most of this century. Essentially the business of diagnosis and treatment is still carried out on two sites: the shop-sized general practice within a mile or two of the patient's home staffed by omni-potential but low-technology doctors and nurses; the hypermarket-sized general hospital within a short bus ride, dealing with everything from childbirth to depressive illness and open heart surgery.

In relation to the future of human genome mapping, John Bell predicts the radical restructuring of the pharmaceutical and biotechnology industries. Yet the very use of the common phrase "the health services *industry*" begs intriguing questions about the future shape and size of all our health-related organisations. Can we reform them in the image of the new clinical science?

In his monograph *Images of Organization*, Gareth Morgan[10] describes the pervasive power of metaphor on the ways in which we think. Metaphor is intrinsic to our use of language, and reveals the feelings and the values beneath the surface of the words we use. Medicine, for example, is much described in military metaphor: doctors *combat* infections caused by *invading* bacteria with *aggressive* treatment, and so on. Ivan Illich,[11] tracing changing medical attitudes through the iconography of the library plates of doctors, noted that before the eighteenth century the doctor was depicted as dancing with the Angel of Death: following the Enlightenment, he is seen no longer dancing with her but struggling – opposing her with shield and sword.

Metaphor at once instructs and discomforts us by its audacious conjunctions, it allows us to see one reality as though it were another, it disrupts expectation with fresh perspectives, it springs the surprises that constitute the discoveries of science, and the revelations of art. The exploration of metaphor constitutes a key tool in the contemporary analysis of art, linguistics, theoretical physics, psychoanalysis, social theory, and much else. Morgan's contribution is to apply such analysis to the theory of organisations. What metaphors of health service organisation are implied by these clinical futures?

Morgan develops an intriguing taxonomy, images of the organisations within which we work that *seem* part of common experience, but are in fact rather *strangely* familiar. The commonest metaphor is the organisation as "machine", with its emphasis on central control, explicit rules, rigid discipline, uniformity, specialisation of functions, and predictability. In essence this finds its apotheosis in early twentieth century engineering mass production. But its antecedents go back at least to Descartes and his notion of mechanical Man.[12]

The current drive to regulate medical practice according to the lights of evidence-based medicine, described earlier, is compatible with the notion of a "health services *industry*", but may well not serve the purposes of the future clinical practice adumbrated here. There are reasons to suggest that organisations shaped by the current values of economy of scale and efficiency may prove incompatible with a medical science that expresses the randomness, complexity, profligacy and environmental sensitivity of our biological natures.

Morgan describes many other metaphors of organisation. A future neuropsychiatry clinic as "bio-organism" would contrast sharply with the contemporary coronary intensive care unit as "machine". In the organisation as bio-organism there would be a deep concern to preserve the *internal* environment, while at the same time discovering ecological niches: contemporary general practices, and in recent years particularly "fund-holders", were rather like that.

In what he calls the organisation as "psychic prison" its members are perpetually trapped by half-suppressed memories of a real or imagined history. Drawing on Jungian imagery, here Morgan suggests that organisational life can be understood in terms of the relationship between fools, magicians, warriors, high priests, lovers, and other symbolic characters. The fierce fights to preserve many of the great London Teaching Hospitals from closure (mooted as part of recent attempts to rationalise London's health services) conjures up just such a metaphor.

Morgan also points out that we are free to reinvent our own images of organisation. For this fusion between organisation and imagination, Morgan coins the term "imaginization". Imaginization suggests that we can perpetually reinvent what appear to be the "givens" of our great institutions. Based on the biotechnology and information technology predicted in the coming chapters, what scenario of health services can be imaginized?

We may begin the reinvention of our great institutions by questioning their appropriateness in terms of size, dominance, and rigid conformity. Poole-Wilson warns of the dangers of reducing the number of independent medical schools and research laboratories, consequent on the drive now to mergers and the creation of very large multidisciplinary research groups, with power and control vested in few hands. He writes: "True innovation may be snuffed out by these monoliths".

In place of the present *hierarchical* arrangements of care, we will have complex *networks* of location and people. It is from web-like images associated with the ecosystem and the internet that the new health-care organisations may derive their structure and function. The drivers for this will include the democratisation of knowledge, powerful software, telecommunications, the personal biosensor woven into the fabric of the body, and the patient-held medical record on a "smart card".

Personnel

The institutions will change, and also the tasks and training of health-care professionals. The march of technology will make it necessary for specialists not only constantly to revise technical knowledge and skills, but radically to "begin again", to acquire quite new skills in mid-career, as the redundancy rates of successive technologies accelerate.

A paradox of advancing bio- and information technology is that while medical science becomes increasingly sophisticated and arcane, the operation of its tools becomes simplified. The use of future technology will not require the same degree of long and in-depth training as that currently required of doctors. Some 50 years ago, Lord Cohen of Birkenhead asserted that the three tasks of the doctor were "diagnosis, diagnosis and diagnosis". Fifty years hence, the primacy of this diagnostic task may well remain. Treatment, however, will be in the hands of a wide range of highly differentiated therapists who will recognise no boundary between what we now call primary and secondary care. Their expertise, orientation and training will develop from that of today's specialist nurses (surgical, medical, paediatric, and psychiatric), from diagnostic radiographers and pharmacists, but also from technologies not yet conceived.

Although the doctor may still be concerned with Lord Cohen's "diagnosis, diagnosis, and diagnosis", the diagnostic task will be transformed. The outline is already clear in current practice. Problem solving at the patient's side (note not *bedside*) will be based on computer interrogated history, data from biosensing monitors, Bayesian computer analysis, and the immediate availability of a second opinion by teleconferencing (to a patient in Bolton, from a specialist in Santa Barbara).

In terms of state-of-the art interventions, patients will wish to go to centres of excellence, and will know where they are. The quality of these centres' performance will in part be a function of the quantity of their cases treated. Catherine Peckham quotes:

Twenty-five years of experience in paediatric cardiac surgery have convinced me that the sickest neonate with severe congenital heart defects could be safely transferred to the other side of the world to be treated in a specialised unit.

The traditional division of labour between general practitioners and hospital-based specialists has resulted in the evolution of two quite distinct diagnostic tasks. That of the specialist is to *reduce* uncertainty, to explore *possibility*, and to marginalise *error*. That of the general practitioner is to mediate between the predicament of the individual and the potential of bioscience: it is to *tolerate* uncertainty, to explore *probability*, and to marginalise *danger*.[13] But the necessity for this previously crucial division must soon be questioned on both technical and moral grounds.

In the future, the patient herself will be enabled to participate much more actively. As the patient assumes this more active role, utilising the open access to biomedical information, will she still need a generalist adviser at the very point of entry into health care? Until recently I assumed that of course she would, that the present-day role of the general practitioner would continue to be a universal and unchanging need in delivering an efficient and humane service. Now I am less certain. It may well be that the twentieth-century roles of the general practitioner as guardian of the patients best interest will come to be seen in quite a different light (paternalistic control rather than caring partisanship) in the next century. Also, it must be admitted that the description of the specialist function in medicine as essentially biomechanical, and that of the general practitioner as essentially psychosocial, was always both an over-simplification, and, for both, something of a canard.

There will be new ways to assist the patient in her decision making. A rich variety of inputs, for example the availability on-line of diagnostic software in the patient's home, may make her initial decisions safe enough. Interrogation by computer is already capable of achieving a more detailed set of data than that resulting from conventional history taking. In future, progress with artificial intelligence will greatly enhance the interpretation of these data. Add to these the data from the biosensing technology described in Chapter 3, and a very powerful clinical problem-solving machine is placed in the patient's own hands. These developments will substantially answer current anxieties about the consequences of direct access to specialist services.

Such a system of self-referral will also address a moral dilemma already troubling the European Parliament.[14] The UK referral system, the convention (as a matter of professional etiquette, not of law) that no consultant specialist will see a patient unless consulted on her behalf by a general practitioner, may be thought to limit iatrogenic damage and contribute to efficiency, but it can also be judged as a gross infringement of the patient's civil liberty.

We can envisage a new web-like system of health care in which the pivotal player is the patient herself. Most initial contacts will be with what I will call socio-nursing professionals operating from small primary units located in high streets and hypermarkets, business and commercial centres, central transport terminals, and schools. From here, but also as easily from the patient's home, direct access to highly specialised facilities will be made possible by the use of telecommunication technology.

The generalist tradition was most completely developed in twentieth century British general practice. It included competence in "multi-paradigm" clinical thinking, in the interpretation of a great diversity of data, in the analysis and presentation of complex moral issues, and in sensitivity to the patient's values and biography. Such competences and habits of thinking will continue to be needed, and integrated into the training of the new socio-nursing profession that I envisage – and also into the training of future specialists. The excellence of the successful specialist has always been marked by an instinctual feeling for the specialness of the patient, which is of the essence of the generalist tradition in medicine. But will there be a need for a specific group of "clinical generalists" in the future?

Precisely because of the advances in technology suggested here, it may become prudent to invent what elsewhere I described as Renaissance physicians,[13] doctors capable of acting as generalist consultants and case managers through all the clinical pathways, and across all the interfaces, of the patient's care. The challenges of creating such a consultancy will be immense, both intellectually and logistically. I suggest that the pressure to invent this New Generalist may come simultaneously from the New Patient and her New Specialist, and it may prove irresistible.

Boundaries

What is portended for the quality of life? Here is a passage about the new human condition, from a 1996 edition of the popular weekly magazine *New Scientist*:

14

You're 55 and it's time to think about having a baby. Luckily your mother was a progressive thinker. When you were a teenager she made sure that you put a few of your eggs into a fertility bank – just in case you were so busy with your career that you put off babies until retirement. That's the way it turned out. Now, thanks to her foresight, you'll be able to have your own child rather than buy someone else's eggs. All that remains is to call up the company's on-line catalogue and choose a sperm donor. Brain-gene therapists are fashionable this year, but since you're a bit of an intellectual yourself, you fancy an Olympic athlete as your child's father . . .

I cannot recall how "futuristic" this passage appeared a mere 2 years ago: today it seems pretty tame stuff. Chapter 7 describes the monitoring of the detailed development of the fetus *in utero*, *in utero* surgery, and the introduction of genetically modified tissue. None of these advances, I think, offers any particularly new challenge to our concept of what it means to be human.

Grimley Evans describes the biological balance struck between the energy devoted to tissue repair (determining the rate at which the organism ages) and that deployed for reproduction (determining the survival of the species). He hints darkly that we may be able to shift the balance pharmacologically, to live longer at the cost of our reproductive drive: an exquisite choice!

More challenging are the implications of xenotransplants discussed by Poole-Wilson in Chapter 6. These may well raise anxieties about the nature of identity similar to those that first appeared with the advent of donor human organ transplants. But the inclusion of a genetically modified pig's heart may soon come to cause no greater perturbation than the ingestion of a genetically modified bacon sandwich.

David Delpys comment: "A particularly exciting development is the research into direct brain–machine interfaces, which although in its infancy, offers great promise for very profoundly disabled people . . .", raises quite another level of disquiet. Particularly if we think about the interface in relation not only to motor function (which he is writing about here) but also to cognitive function; and not only as a treatment for brain damage, but as an enhancement and extension of healthy function.

In contemplating the possibilities of direct brain–machine interfaces, it is precisely the nature of the "directness" that shocks. As I type these lines using the word-processing programme of my desktop computer, I am able to click on the icon of my archived files and rediscover lost "unremembered" material from previous essays (that is how I came across the passage from *New Scientist*, quoted above). Part of my memory is now silicon based, and I am engaged at the cognitive level in a brain–machine interface. This feels distinctly different from the brain–machine interface at work when I listen (as I do now, while writing this) to a Handel aria on my CD player. It is the future *incorporation* of machine or cell xenotransplant into the substance of my body that raises questions about the bounds of remaining human.

Contemplation of a brain–machine interface suggests that there will be no future boundary discernible between the use of biotechnologies in the prevention and cure of disease, and their use as instruments of recreation. Drugs developed to counter the ravages of Alzheimer's disease may be adapted to enhance the function of memory in the healthy brain. Iversen describes the growing field of "psychoneuroimmunology" and predicts the advent of drugs that will permanently set the brain's control of body weight to a preferred figure, creating "a new industry rivalling the diet business in size".

The recent introduction of finasteride for male pattern baldness, is a current example of therapy at the interface with cosmetics. Sildenafil, as a treatment for erectile dysfunction, has taken the world of pharmaceutical marketing by storm, and is the embodiment (also in the literal sense) of the growing medicalisation of life. Such innovations will increasingly pose questions for health services about what is and is not an entitlement, about the scope of private and public health-care assurance.

But beyond the question of cost and who pays, there are more intractable questions about the limits of medicine, about where society will draw the line between what is deemed health need, and lifestyle wish. The current debates about the availability of *in vitro* fertilisation as a NHS entitlement are but storm petrels. The new technology will compound rather than resolve these dilemmas. Yet the wide democratisation of knowledge must eventually totally breach the gate of what was once "the secret garden" of medicine.

Most of our authors have raised questions not about our future integrity as human *individuals* in the light of the new technologies (which appears not to cause them much anxiety), but about the future integrity of our human *societies* (which does). They examine the relationship between two of the key principles of the health service in the UK, and the conflict between them. The first principle is excellence – the imperative to deliver to the patient the best of contemporary medicine. Excellence, of course, is not simply a matter of technological but also of cultural values.

Grimley Evans sees a peculiarly English virtue with regard to the stoic acceptance of mortality, and warns that before long ". . . we shall be in earshot of alien voices bewailing their mortality". But he also observes (surely a mordant aside on genetic engineering) that there may be few limits to our pursuit of excellence: "Serial monogamy will no doubt continue to grow in popularity, and older, fitter (and richer) men will have the opportunity to revert to the social habits of our primate ancestors in breeding from a succession of younger consorts."

The second principle is equity – the ethic of delivering fair shares to all the members of society, based not on ability to pay, but on clinical need. The needs of vulnerable groups – the children, the old, the poor, those with profound and enduring disabilities – are all addressed. Most of our writers take a global view of equity, and some of the statistics they quote are deeply disturbing. Catherine Peckham writes, "Centuries separate the lives and fates of children living today in different parts of the globe". Sikora points to a similarly grim contrast between the control of cancer in the developed countries, and the Third World. It is clear that just as the technical boundaries of our "humanness" will continue to challenge our imaginations, so the political boundaries of health care will continue to challenge our sense of justice.

Envoi

While no clear consensus emerges, or should be expected from clinical science, about the specific political governance of the NHS, or of international health-care policy, what does emerge very clearly is a powerful and shared sense of optimism in the power of medical science and technology to improve the lot of the individual, of society, and of the global performance of health services. And, I think, a commitment to the founding principles (not least the principle of social fairness and inclusivity) of the NHS whose fiftieth anniversary this book was written to celebrate.

Clinical science has, in the century that now closes, delivered much to the quality of the life of the common man, and to the achievement of a more equitable society. Surely this is the compelling evidence from the progress so far in anaesthesia, vaccines, antibiotics, and so on. The moral test ahead, touched on by all our authors, will be the future access to all the services foreshadowed here, by all our citizens. Again, there is cause for cautious optimism. The history of the motor car, the refrigerator, and currently the mobile phone, suggests that technological innovation cannot be socially controlled, or succeed commercially, only as toys for the privileged few.

Freeman Dyson distinguishes between two contrasting styles of technological development.[1] The first, relatively unsuccessful either in making money for its backers, or in improving the lot of society, he describes as "Napoleonic". The second, which he describes as "Tolstoyan", succeeds both commercially and societally. Napoleonic technology is vast, is rigid and controlling in its development, and is usually driven by political imperatives. Tolstoyan technology is driven by the enthusiasm of its inventors, is flexible and responsive, and is tested by the market not the ideology. The Zeppelins, nuclear energy and the IBM mainframes were, he claims, Napoleonic: the aeroplane and the internet were Tolstoyan. The heart transplant programme is Tolstoyan; the mass cervical cytology screening programme, Napoleonic. It is not the size and complexity of the technology that determines comparison with Napoleon and Tolstoy, but the way in which it is politicised, developed and deployed. Much that is here adumbrated, seems reassuringly Tolstoyan.

Most modern thinkers seem to have rejected a determinist analysis of history. In *Virtual History*,[15] a collection of essays by a number of academic historians about "counterfactual history", Niall Ferguson points out that at every point in history the possibility existed that things might have gone differently from what ensued. The essays draw on the rigorous examination of contemporary documentation to illustrate the un-inevitability of past events: counterfactual histories are created, based closely on the documentary evidence of the day, that plot the avoidance of the Civil War in the 1630s and so the survival of the monarchy under Charles; the success of Home Rule for a British United Ireland in 1912; a decision in Britain's self-interest to "stand aside" and not go to war with the Kaiser's Germany in 1914.

Such a view of the past assures us that there are no pre-determined futures, no bio-medical "discoveries" waiting patiently out there in the next millennium, for us to arrive at the appropriate time and claim them. There is a sense in these essays not of scientific discovery, but of contingent creativity and invention. This book is probably safest read as a counterfactual history of clinical medicine's future.

At the outset I noted that one way or another all of our authors, enjoined to look ahead further than their rigorous habits of thought made comfortable, warned against the dangers of forecasting, or its more misleading and sinister counterfeit, prediction. Poole-Wilson invokes George Eliot ("Of all errors prophecy is the most pernicious"), and I began with WH Auden's knowing disclaimer. In defence of our attempt to peer into the mists of the day after tomorrow I end by quoting Auden again, from another poem in which he offers a further comment on the paradox of an unknowable future, and our compulsion to read it. The poem is helpfully titled "Leap Before You Look":

> The sense of danger must not disappear:
> The way is certainly both short and steep,
> However gradual it looks from here;
> Look if you like, but you will have to leap.

References

1 Dyson F. *Imagined worlds*. Harvard, 1997.
2 Kuhn T. *The structure of scientific revolutions*, 1997.
3 Dally A. Thalidomide: was the tragedy preventable? *Lancet* 1998, 351: 1197–99.
4 Quoted in Roszack T. *The cult of information*, 1994
5 Comroe JH Jr. The clouded crystal ball. *Am Rev Resp Dis* 1975; 111: 795–802.
6 Bronowski J. *Science and human values*. London, 1961.
7 Evidence-based Medicine Working Group, Evidence based medicine: a new approach to teaching the practice of medicine. *JAMA* 1992; 268: 2420–5.
8 Wilkinson RG. Income distribution and life expectancy. *Br Med J* 1992; 304: 165–8.
9 Nesse RM, Williams GC. *Evolution and Healing*, 1995.
10 Morgan G. *Images of organisation*, 1986.
11 Illich I. *Medical nemesis*, 1970.
12 Descartes R. *L'homme machine*, 1748.
13 Marinker M. *The end of general practice. The 1995 Bayliss Lecture*. London: PPP.
14 Marinker M. The referral system. *J R Coll Gen Pract* 1988; 38: 487–91.
15 Ferguson N. *Virtual history*. London, 1997.

2 The human genome

John Bell

Introduction

Every 50 years, a breakthrough in basic science feeds through to provide a major change in the practice of clinical medicine. Some of these advances have emanated from basic biological science, such as the revolution in microbiology at the end of the nineteenth century that eventually led to the development of effective antimicrobial therapy and the successful assault on many infectious diseases. On a more modest scale, basic advances in immunology have led to significant changes in our understanding of and therapy for immune-mediated disease. In other cases, developments in the basic science had been in non-biological areas. No one would argue about the impact of the silicon chip and microprocessors on modern western medicine in the second half of the twentieth century. Progressing many basic science developments to the bedside has sometimes proved slow, with major advances in science impacting on clinical practice only after 20–50 years. Few would question that recent developments in genetics will prove to be the most significant scientific advances of the current era and it is inevitable that this will eventually feed through to affect many, if not all, of clinical medicine. As with infectious disease, genetics is fundamentally involved with disease pathogenesis, but in addition it is responsible for many aspects of response to therapy and disease outcomes. As a result, the impact of genetics on medicine may well prove to be greater than any previous scientific advance.

The timing of advances in human genetics coincides with a crisis in clinical practice and health-care systems that have evolved in the last 50 years. Financial, demographic and philosophical factors will all precipitate dramatic changes in medicine in the next decade. The limitations in our current practice of medicine are many and they will require substantial changes in our approach to patients with disease if medicine is to continue to thrive into the next millennium. The solution to many of the problems may be found as the impact of human genetics is felt in the clinical sector.

The limitations of current clinical practice

Although clinical medicine has made tremendous progress over the last 50 years, there are clearly substantial limitations to medicine as it is currently practised. Not only has the overall burden of disease increased due to demographic changes, but the extent of chronic disease and our ability to manage it to reduce disability is clearly limited. Contrasted with the considerable success we have had in managing some acute illnesses, such as the major infectious diseases, little progress has been made in preventing or treating diseases such as diabetes, asthma, athritis, or cancer. The explanations for this lack of success are many but they include the major problems discussed below.

Late application of therapy

Most disorders of adult life are preceded by a prolonged presymptomatic period. Vascular disease is known to begin early in life, long before the disease becomes symptomatic, while symptomatic Type II diabetes may be preceded by many years of abnormal glucose tolerance. Much of current medical practice is applied to resolving the problems associated with symptomatic disease, late in the natural history of most of these disorders. Only in a few circumstances have drugs been applied to treat presymptomatic individuals in an attempt to prevent the end-stage sequelae of these abnormalities. The treatment of hypertension and hyperlipidaemia are two examples of where such early therapy has had a profound impact on the management of vascular disease. These problems are also highlighted by the problems associated with screening programmes for diseases such as breast or cervical cancer. These attempts to identify individuals early in the course of disease have been hampered by the difficulties of screening a large segment of the population without stratification. The ability to treat disease early to alter its natural history, rather than treating end-stage disease, ultimately requires methods for early presymptomatic diagnosis and early targeted and safe therapy.

Diseases are defined by the phenotype not their mechanisms

The failure to define diseases and their mechanisms has profound implications on the ability to anticipate the natural history and adequately treat diseases, utilising information about their biochemical basis rather than simply their phenotype. For example, diseases such as diabetes may result from many distinct mechanisms that raise blood sugar while asthma may occur as the result of multiple different causes of bronchospasm or atopy. Understanding and defining the mechanism of disease will permit a clearer definition of these disorders and will have implications for a more precise prediction of their natural history, and more precise targeting of appropriate therapies. At the present time the tendency is to "lump" disorders together based on phenotype criteria, which greatly limits the ability to adequately manage each patient. In the future it will be necessary to split chronic disease phenotypes into different mechanistically defined categories to facilitate the appropriate application of clinical practice.

Therapy is used in heterogeneous groups of patients, resulting in a wide range of therapeutic responses

At the present time therapeutic interventions are used in chronic disease with the knowledge that patients may respond beneficially to particular drugs, but also may either fail to respond or may show serious toxicity to the agent. It is not possible, at present, to predict which category individual patients will fall into. A range of different factors are likely to contribute to this variation in response to therapy. The first and most important variation will be that patients treated for the same disease may have fundamentally different pathophysiological mechanisms (see above). This will mean they will respond differently to therapy and appropriate therapy may be different among the different groups. A second possibility for variation in response to therapy relates to differences in drug metabolism or the biotransformation of drugs in different individuals.

Finally there are a cascade of proteins involved in drug action, each of which may be variable in a population and which may determine differential response to a particular therapeutic agent. These three factors, referred to as pharmacogenomics, will be clearly defined in the near future, and will provide important information for those managing patients with chronic disease.

The common theme in all of these factors that limit current clinical practice is that we know too little about the variation in population that leads to differential disease susceptibility, disease mechanisms, and drug response, and it is not possible to accurately identify those at risk before symptoms occur. An understanding of the basics of variation will inevitably lead to an ability to predict disease risk and individualise therapy, with very considerable improvements in outcome and cost–benefit ratios. These developments will arise from the application of modern molecular genetics to the problem of human disease. The remainder of this chapter will discuss how modern human molecular genetics is likely to rapidly provide us with the information we need to implement changes and correct the deficiencies outlined above.

Genes, polymorphisms and mutations

There are about 100 000 expressed genes in the human genome, many of which have now been sequenced and are available to those studying disease genetics. These genes are made up of strands of deoxyribonucleic acids (DNA). The bases cytosine, thymine, guanine, and adenine are linked to five carbon sugars that carry phosphate groups and these nucleotides are joined in tandem to form strands of DNA. Within a code generated by nucleotides in a DNA strand, there lies the instructions for the synthesis of proteins from amino acids. The sequence of each triplet of nucleotides in a coding sequence encodes a single amino acid, this code is transmitted through messenger RNA to ribosomes where polypeptide chains are created from amino acids. When folded, these produce the proteins that are responsible for most cellular structures and functions. Variation in most aspects of human biology is therefore associated with changes in triple code of DNA and this arises predominantly by mutation. These mutations can lead to the transition of one nucleotide to another, changing the code and the amino acid, or can lead to the insertion or deletion of base pairs, leading to a break in the frame of the triplet code and hence an abnormal or shortened protein. Some of these modifications are silent, while others have important functional effects on the encoded protein. Where function is changed, selection can lead to increased frequency in the population or to an elimination of detrimental variants. The mutation and selection of DNA variants, because of a conferred advantage in the host, underlies all our current concepts of evolution. The diversity generated by such DNA variance accounts for much of the variation seen in human populations, and accounts for much of the variation in disease susceptibility and response to therapy in the population.

In addition to DNA variance that alters coding sequence, variation in non-coding regions of DNA can also have important effects in mediating changes in physiology or disease pathogenesis. Sequences upstream of coding regions are responsible for the regulation of transcription of proteins and variation in these regions can determine the levels of proteins present in individual cells or tissues. Similarly, variation in non-coding regions can alter the splicing pattern of cells and produce significant variance in protein structure. Again these DNA variations can have profound functional effects and can in some cases be selected because of their beneficial effects in individuals and in populations.

Against a background of mutations occurring throughout the genome, particular DNA variants are selected because of beneficial effects. One of the best examples of such selection of DNA variation occurs in molecules responsible for determining the immune response to infectious pathogens. The highly variable HLA alleles have been extensively selected for their ability to present pathogen peptides to the immune system. The HLA allele HLABw53, for example, protects West African children from severe malaria, and has hence been periodically selected in that population where it has high allele frequency. It is less common in regions where malaria selection has not been present.

Such DNA variants are referred to as polymorphisms. Their frequency is usually controlled by a balance between beneficial effect and detrimental effect of these polymorphisms in populations. Often the detrimental effect of such alleles may be an increased liability of another disease. This is important in our understanding of polymorphism and its role in human disease, as many of the DNA variants that account for disease susceptibility in populations are polymorphisms that have been selected because of some beneficial effect they confer on individuals. The concept of "bad" genes in the context of common human disease is an erroneous one. Most, if not all of the DNA variants that account for disease susceptibility carry with them beneficial effects and hence have been important for survival in another set of environmental conditions.

Genes and disease

Lessons from single genes

It is clear that the understanding of genetic factors responsible for fully penetrant single gene disorders has enhanced our ability to detect and eventually treat these disorders. The majority of these diseases fall within the domain of the clinical genetics community and the early successes in defining the genetic basis of diseases such as muscular dystrophy, Huntingdon's disease, myotonic dystrophy, fragile X syndrome and cystic fibrosis has already led to a revolution in our ability to predict, screen and understand these diseases. The power of human genetics in defining the molecular basis of these diseases could have been relatively easily predicted because of their simple inheritance patterns. The impact of this body of knowledge on preventative medical care is likely to be small, however, largely due to the infrequency of these disorders in the population. Nevertheless, a few highly penetrant single gene disorders do occur at a sufficiently high frequency to have a substantial public health implication. One such example is hereditary haemochromatosis. The gene mutation responsible for this disease has been characterised and involves the mutation of cysteine involved in an intrachain disulphide bond in the $\alpha3$ domain of an HLA-like molecule on chromosome 6. The cloning and characterisation of this DNA variant and the subsequent characterisation of the molecule mutated in this disorder has provided remarkable insights into the disease. These observations, likely to provide an understanding of the molecular basis of iron loading in such patients, will provide an opportunity to screen for individuals at risk for this disease and provide early intervention in the form of venesection to prevent the long-term sequelae, and finally provide evolutionary insights as to why an allele responsible for iron loading will have been selected to such high frequency in human populations.

Genetic contributions to common disease

Compared to the infrequent single gene disorders, understanding the genetic contribution to common human disease provides a considerably greater opportunity to impact on health care in the future. While the mapping of single gene disorders provided the basic paradigm for tracking genes, the greatest challenge was to come from attempting to identify genes involved in diseases where multiple genetic factors were involved and interact with environmental determinants. The range of diseases which can be tackled using such genetic approaches is extremely broad, accounting for most of the major causes of morbidity and mortality in human populations (Table 2.1). Many common diseases are well recognised to have a strong genetic susceptibility component while other diseases, such as the infectious diseases, have only recently emerged as disorders where susceptibility and response to infection is heavily determined by genetic susceptibility factors.

Several fundamental differences between this form of genetics

Table 2.1 Examples of common diseases with strong genetic susceptibility

Cardiovascular	Ischaemic heart disease†
	Peripheral vascular disease*
	Hypertrophic cardiomyopathy†
	Dilated cardiomyopathy
	Long Q–T syndrome†
	Rheumatic vascular disease*
	Pulmonary thromboembolism†
Respiratory	Asthma†
	Chronic obstructive airways disease
Gastroenterology	Inflammatory bowel disease*
	Chronic active liver disease*
	Coeliac disease†
	Haemochromatosis†
Endocrine	Type 2 diabetes†
	Type 1 diabetes†
	Autoimmune thyroid disease†
	Polycystic ovary syndrome*
	Osteoporosis*
Rheumatology	Rheumatoid arthritis†
	Ankylosing spondylitis†
	Reiter's syndrome†
	Osteoarthritis*
	SLE*
Nephrology	Glomerulonephritis*
	Renal stone disease†
	Gout†
	Renal tubular disease†
Oncology	Breast cancer†
	Colon cancer†
	Ovarian cancer
	Prostate cancer*
Neurology	Alzheimer's disease†
	Myasthenia gravis†
	Multiple sclerosis*
	Epilepsy†
	Migraine†
	Motor neuron disease†
Psychiatry	Schizophrenia*
	Manic depressive psychosis*
	Anxiety disorders*
	Alcoholism†

* Locus identified by linkage analysis.
† Gene and DNA variant cloned.

and that seen in many single gene disorders have emerged. Most importantly, it is clear that the genetic susceptibility responsible for most common diseases are genetic factors which have been selected in populations for their beneficial effects. So, for example, a host of immune response genes and immunologically important polymorphisms clearly dictate susceptibility to infectious pathogens as well as to autoimmune diseases. These polymorphisms have largely been selected for their beneficial effects against particular pathogens. Similarly, it is likely that many of the genes involved in metabolic disorders such as diabetes, obesity and cardiovascular disease may have been selected because of their abilities to provide individuals with an advantage during times of famine (i.e. "thrifty genotype"). These polymorphoric genetic variants are therefore not truly disease genes, but often have some beneficial phenotypical characteristic associated with their expression, hence they have been selected in high frequency in the population.

There have already been considerable advances in the characterisation of genes involved in susceptibility to many common human diseases. A pattern has emerged which suggested many of these diseases, such as breast cancer, hypertension and diabetes, represent multiple different disorders, each resulting in the phenotype which is the basis for the clinical diagnosis. This highlights one of the previously highlighted limitations in current clinical practice, that diseases are commonly defined using simple phenotypic criteria with no understanding of mechanism. Genetics is rapidly revealing the difficulties with this phenotypic approach, in that most common diseases appear to have several distinct mechanisms, each with distinct, natural features and each with different optimal therapies.

Almost all of the major common disorders include a subset of patients in whom genetic susceptibility is dominant. This sort of genetic disease is relatively tractable and many such genes have now been localised. They often provide significant examples of how a particular phenotype can be created from a range of different mechanisms, and are easier to understand mechanistically because environment appears to play little role. The breast cancer genes *BRCA1/BRCA2* are examples of highly penetrant disease susceptibility loci, as are the *MODY* loci for Type 2 diabetes, *MODY 1, 2,* and *3*. In general, however, these highly penetrant disease loci contribute little to the overall burden of disease, accounting for between 5% and 10% of disease frequency in the population. Nevertheless, for extremely common diseases, such as colon cancer, the ability to detect individuals at risk by screening *APC* genes and *HNPCC* genes would allow for detection of up to 10% of colon cancer in the population. Given the frequency of this disease, this would have a very significant impact on the approach to this disease in the future.

Perhaps the most important outcome of genetic mapping studies in common disease to date has been that they provide a much clearer understanding of the biological events that may lead to distortions in physiology that produce morbidity and mortality in the population. In Type 2 diabetes, for example, there is now clear evidence for abnormalities in the glucokinase glucostat being responsible for some forms of the disease, while other forms of the disease are the result of insulin receptor mutations or mutations in transcription factors which may be expressed in the beta cell or the liver. These have provided whole new insights into the mechanisms of these disorders and, ultimately, this is likely to have an impact on our understanding of the natural history of the various subtypes of disease, their optimum therapy, and potentially the complications associated with each of them.

Molecular genetics and a new taxonomy for common disease

What is emerging from the current studies of common disease genetics is that extensive heterogeneity exists under the umbrella of current diagnostic categories. Such "lumping" has clearly impeded our ability to provide optimum medical care to many individuals. Individuals have been treated as if they have the same disease when in fact, biologically speaking, they have totally different disorders, but simply share some particular phenotypic outcome. In the past it has proved extremely difficult to dissect individual disease subtypes in a precise fashion. Histopathology has been used as a rather limited tool to define pathological subtypes of disease, but the constraints on such morphological assessments are clear. Only in the infectious diseases has a century of microbiology and virology provided us with clear insights into these mechanisms. For example, hepatitis has in the past been a clinical phenotype that encompassed a range of patients suffering from non-obstructive forms of jaundice but who had widely differing natural histories, prognoses, and for whom no clear therapy has been identified. The ability to dissect the mechanisms responsible for hepatitis, partic- ularly the various viruses involved (hepatitis A, B, C, E) has helped different clinical syndromes with differing natural histories. Perhaps most interesting is that therapies which are now believed to have some therapeutic effect in one subtype or another (i.e., alpha interferon in hepatitis C) would have been shown to be ineffective if all forms of hepatitis had been lumped together without a clear understanding of their mechanisms. A similar scenario confronts us in most of the other non-infectious diseases, whereby normal therapies are doomed to fail because of the heterogeneity underlying a particular disease phenotype, and where a clinician's ability to predict outcome or manage a patient reliably is severely impeded by the lack of diagnostic precision.

It is clear that an improved understanding of the various mechanisms of disease will provide huge opportunities for better patient diagnosis and management, and that is likely to arise from the substantial molecular genetic efforts to define disease pathways in many common disorders. This is particularly interesting in the context of the apparent variation in disease frequency and pattern in different ethnic populations. Hypertension, for example, is well known to be particularly severe in black populations and is often ACE inhibitor resistant. Similarly, Type 2 diabetes is found at dramatic frequencies of 15–50% in particular ethnic populations, particularly those in Asia and the South Pacific. These variations are likely to arise from differences in gene frequencies and genetic polymorphisms responsible for these phenotypes in different populations, and may have profound implications on how such individuals should be managed clinically. Overall, an understanding of the biochemical pathways involved in a disease process will allow us to move to a new disease taxonomy, with disease being diagnosed and managed rationally, based on mechanism rather than on haphazard notions based on phenotypic criteria.

Genetics and new opportunities for therapy

Targets

A clear understanding of genetic susceptibility could provide the information necessary to contract to development and targeting of new therapies. Genetics is very likely to provide a range of new targets which will allow a more rational and rapid approach to drug design. Genetic approaches have provided the pharmaceutical industry with a wealth of new targets against which to design drugs. Genetics may provide the industry with the means to identify targets implicated in major biochemical pathways involved in

29

disease pathogenesis and will also identify control points on biochemical pathways that may be particularly amenable to interventions. For example the discovery of leptin, using genetic techniques, has opened up a whole pathway with many targets for the development of drugs for obesity. Whether individual disease genes emerge as useful targets in the future may be less important than the fact that the pharmaceutical industry will be pursuing new therapies based on careful and rational understanding of disease processes, rather than by allowing them compound screening.

Pharmacogenomics

Perhaps the first widespread important clinical application of human molecular genetics will be in identifying individuals capable of responding to particular therapeutic interventions, or identifying those unlikely to respond or likely to suffer toxicity due to a particular agent. The wide diversity of response to individual drugs is well recognised by clinicians and pharmaceutical companies alike. In the course of drug development many therapeutic agents provide promising phase 2 clinical data, only to fail at phase 3 clinical trials. Such results are likely to be due to the fact that the patient populations used for these studies are heterogeneous. The inability to select homogeneous patient populations has meant the drug development process has become both risky and expensive. Similar experiences are common in a clinic. Patients respond with substantial variability to most antihypertension medications, and the inability to predict responsiveness leads to poor blood pressure control or treatment with several agents in many patients. Similar problems exist with the use of most therapies in patient populations, all arising because of genetic variation. In addition, drug toxicity has proved to be a major limiting factor in modern medicine. Some effective agents have toxicity in individuals that prevent their use in a responding population, and who cannot be identified from those suffering toxicity. Similarly, relatively rare but important but sometimes fatal toxic effects are important for drugs that are widely used. The ability to identify individuals at risk of such severe toxicity would greatly enhance the practice of clinical medicine.

There are three general ways in which our understanding of genetics is likely to impact on our use of therapeutics in the future. The first area relates to polymorphisms of enzymes involved in the biotransformation of drugs. These enzymes play a central role in modifying compounds we are exposed to in the environment and have therefore been selected extensively in human populations and many contain substantial degrees of genetic polymorphisms. The effects of such biotransformation enzyme polymorphisms have been recognised for many years and have had a significant impact on a range of drugs evaluated as early as the 1960s when debrisoquine toxicity was shown to be the result of polymorphism in the cytochrome P450 enzyme CYP2D6, and acetylator polymorphisms were shown to account for the variation in handling agents such as isoniazid or hydralazine. Molecular techniques have demonstrated that many such enzymes are polymorphic (Table 2.2). Toxicity from drugs is often related to drug metabolism and its variation in the population and hence the ability to identify the DNA variants responsible for these effects, and to predict metabolism and clinical outcomes, is likely to have a profound effect on the way new drugs are both developed and applied in practice.

A second important mechanism for the more precise and accurate application of therapy will be the definition of disease based on genetic mechanisms rather than phenotypes. Individuals who might suffer from totally different forms of hypertension (i.e., one associated with abnormal salt handling versus another associated with catecholamines) are likely to be differentially responsive to therapies directed at such mechanisms. Understanding, genetically and mechanistically, the factors responsible for the disease susceptibility will undoubtedly lead to substantial further precision in the use of drugs.

Table 2.2   Allele frequencies for certain polymorphic CYP450 enzymes in Caucasians

Enzyme polymorphism		Frequency
CYP2A6	Consensus	78%
CYP2A6v1		17%
CYP2A6v2		7%
CYP2C9*1	Consensus	79%
CYP2C9*2		12%
CYP2C9*3		9%
CYP2D6	Consensus	65%
CYP2D6A		4%
CYP2D6B		10%
CYP2D6C		4%

Adapted from C.W. Wolf and 'Pharmacogenomics' (Scrip, 1998)

A third and very important application of genetics, clinical pharmacology, will be the identification of variation in drug targets and molecules associated with them. It is already recognised that many of the common drug targets such as beta adrenoceptors, 5HT receptors, and angiotensin receptors, and in many cases their associated signalling molecules, show polymorphism in the population. Some of these variants have been demonstrated to have important effects on the response or toxicity associated with drugs that utilise them as targets. It is likely that many such polymorphisms will be found and will explain a range of responses in a population to every individual therapy currently available. If such polymorphisms can be shown to predict response then they are likely to be used as an adjunct in everyday clinical practice for the selection of appropriate therapy for different individuals. This important area has only recently been accessible for study through the availability of large sequence databases and extensive characterisation of simple nucleotype polymorphisms in such genomes. It is likely to dictate both drug development and clinical practice extensively in the future.

Genetics and clinical practice

Individualisation of medical practice

One of the clear limitations in current practice is that patients are grouped together because of a particular phenotypic feature, and are then managed using standard protocols. Recently this has been institutionalised in the form of practice guidelines for individual complaints. Beneficial as these approaches have been in the past, they clearly fail to address the central issue in modern medical practice, and that is that very few patients are likely to be truly identical either in the nature of their disease, the presence of particular disease modifiers that alter the response to particular disease insults, or in their response to therapy. As a result, clinical practice has proved to be crude and only sometimes effective. The huge variation in individuals has made the task of applying medical care efficiently across large cohorts of patients difficult because of the wide variation in the genes that relate to or modify a disease phenotype.

Although large randomised controlled trials have become the gold standard for validation of effective therapeutic interventions, the lack of diagnostic precision at entry to such trials means that patient subpopulations, with different disease mechanisms or pharmacogenetic features, will be obscured by the heterogeneity of the overall patient population. Valid active therapy is undoubtedly overlooked by such protocols but they remain the only robust mechanism for currently evaluating therapy. Their utility would be greatly improved and refined if the populations studied at least suffered from the same disease.

As medical care advances, it will be necessary to increasingly recognise this genetic variation, characterise it, and then utilise it by increasing the individualisaton of therapy. This need not provide excessive costs to any health-care system. Given that genetic variants will be easily and inexpensively detected in the relatively near future (see below), it is likely that the information will be available to take such decisions on an individual basis. The resources that are wasted by applying therapies which have no effect or are toxic in some individuals, and the efforts made attempting to treat disease using one mechanistic paradigm when the patient is in fact suffering from a phenocopy of the disease should provide ample leeway to introduce such individualisation of therapy without substantially adding cost. The current system is ineffective because of lack of precision, and if that precision can be gleaned effectively without substantial added cost then the economic benefits are likely to be real.

An additional commercial benefit will be that the cost of drug development is likely to fall. New therapies will be available because of the targets created by genetic technologies. Drug development programmes are more likely to achieve success because of appropriate patient selection and stratification. The utilisation of such genetic definition is likely to be actively encouraged by health-care providers, who are unlikely to be willing to apply drugs in populations where they may be beneficial in only a minority of patients.

Diagnostics as an adjunct to therapy

One of the important aspects of the field of genetics and clinical medicine is that genetic diagnosis is likely to be used in the future as an extremely important tool in the management of all patients. If therapy is going to be utilised in a rational way and if patients are going to be properly categorised before being provided with appropriate advice and therapy, then rapid and efficient diagnostic methods will need to be available. A revolution is occurring in this particular aspect of medical instrumentation in that it is now possible to detect relatively large numbers of single nucleotide polymorphisms simultaneously, using a range of new technologies.

There is now an increasingly powerful international programme to detect the variation that exists within the human genome. The DNA sequence of an entire human genome is likely to be available within the next 5 years, but more importantly as many as 100 000 single nucleotide polymorphisms are likely to be detected over the same timeframe. Some of these polymorphisms will be in noncoding sequences but may be in strong linkage disequilibrium with polymorphisms in coding sequences that are important functionally. This set of polymorphisms is likely to provide a handle on many of the important genetic determinants of disease susceptibility and response to therapy that exist in the population. At the present time, techniques for typing such polymorphisms are slow and laborious. If genetic diagnostics is likely to be widely applied in clinical practice, it is essential that relatively low cost technology is available for typing large numbers of polymorphisms in parallel. The number of DNA variants that will need to be tested in any individual is likely to be large over their lifetime of health care and as a result a systematic in parallel approach to typing polymorphisms may prove to be the most effective. At present single nucleotide polymorphisms (SNPs) are being typed using conventional slab gel technologies or more recently capilliary electrophoresis arrays. These permit a relatively high throughput of polymorphisms but have nowhere near the capability that will be required to detect thousands or tens of thousands of polymorphisms simultaneously. Two new technologies provide the possibility of this in the future. The first of these are microarrays which use oligonucleotides attached in arrays to glass slides or chips. Hybridization of amplified DNA sequences to these oligonucleotides provide information on single nucleotide variation with sufficient redundancy to provide accurate results. Many tens of thousands and eventually hundreds of thousands of oligonucleotides will be available on a single chip, allowing for many single nucleotide polymorphisms to be typed simultaneously for an individual. This raises the possibility that an individual will have their genotyping performed on cord blood and the data on these polymorphisms stored for all future use by medical practitioners. Given the potential impact of genetics on health care over a lifetime, such an approach is likely to be very cost effective. This technology is progressing rapidly with substantial commercial support and it is likely that it will be available for systematic use within the next 2 years. A similarly powerful technology involves mass spectroscopy which should permit the detection of large numbers of single nucleotide polymorphisms with a high degree of accuracy, again in parallel. This technology has not been as well developed but may prove to be as powerful as microarrays in the long term.

If genetic diagnostics are to be used at all stages of medical activity, i.e. for identifying individuals who would benefit from screening, for refining a diagnosis based on mechanisms, and for identifying response for toxicity to a range of therapies, such systematic approaches to genetic typing will be necessary. If genetics is used to identify populations that are particularly responsive to therapy by the pharmaceutical industry prior to the licencing of such agents, it is likely that such genetic testing will accompany regulatory approval for new drugs, and if this is the case it will force the implementation of genetics very rapidly into the clinic.

Genetic stratification

The use of genetics in either selective populations or widely across the population will in the future be necessary to ensure that health care is being directed at those at most risk of individual diseases and outcomes. At present most population screening programmes are acquired generically across particular age groups in an attempt to identify individuals with early disease. The success of programmes such as the breast cancer screening and cervical cancer screening programmes has been limited, because individuals at a particularly high risk of these disorders are managed in the same way as those with no risks. The lack of patient stratification means that significant numbers of low-risk individuals are exposed to the possibility of false-positive results, while high-risk individuals with disease may be identified. Similar criticisms could be made of virtually all existing screening programmes, which are pursued with considerable expense and effort within most health-care systems.

In addition to providing improved methods for identifying individuals at risk of diseases which are subjected to screening tests, genetics may also provide an opportunity to identify relatively small subsets of very high-risk individuals who may benefit from early treatment. The concept of treatment in high-risk individuals has been pioneered through the management of diseases such as hypertension and hypercholesterolaemia. These interventions have validated the concept that early intervention may have important therapeutic benefits if individuals at sufficiently high risk of disease can be identified. The great power of genetic testing is that it identifies such individuals before they have become symptomatic, thus permiting early therapy. This is a central issue in modern clinical practice, as most of our interventions occur at a late stage in disease, often after disability has begun. The ability to intervene early in a large number of diseases may dramatically alter our abilities to reduce disability in the population, and reduce our dependence on intensive resuscitation in individuals with end-stage disease.

One can imagine already how genetics might be applied to further refine our ability to use presymptomatic therapies effectively. It is recognised that the risk of myocardial infarction falls throughout the entire range of cholesterol. Cholesterol-lowering agents are utilised predominantly in individuals with extremes of the phenotype, as it is in this population that the benefits are most cost effective. Individuals with cholesterol levels in the normal range provide a poor cost–benefit ratio unless individuals can be identified with particularly high risks of developing myocardial infarction in this group. Secondary prevention studies have shown that reduction of cholesterol in individuals who had a myocardial infarction provide some benefit. Similarly, one would predict that primary prevention studies of individuals who have significant risk factors, either environmental (smoking) and/or substantial other genetic risk factors for ischaemic heart disease are likely to benefit considerably from cholesterol-lowering therapy, even if their cholesterols are not elevated. Many such opportunities to intervene in presymptomatic patients are likely to arise, particularly if the pharmaceutical industry is confident that risk factor prediction using genetics will allow them to intervene effectively in early stage disease. Diseases such as Alzheimer's disease will be optimal targets for this sort of approach.

The ethics and practice of genetic testing

Predictive testing versus risk factor detection

Predictive testing

There is considerable confusion about the relative role of genetic testing in highly penetrant genetic disorders compared to the identification of genetic factors that confer increased (or reduced) risk of particular diseases. The conventional paradigm established by clinical geneticists is around highly penetrant single gene disorders where the identification of a particular DNA variant is a highly reliable predictor of outcome. Rules for testing have developed around this model, with particular concern about ethical and consent issues. Counselling has played an important role in the management of patients undergoing this form of predictive testing which can relatively accurately provide information about individual risk. This area of genetic testing is likely to undergo substantial changes in the near future. The reason for these changes is that the magnitude of the problem has grown considerably. In particular, with the identification of highly penetrant genes in diseases such as breast cancer and colon cancer, there will be an urgent requirement for the development of testing services for high-risk populations, and perhaps eventually for entire population cohorts, for the detection of these DNA variants. This is particularly true with colon cancer where prophylactic measures are feasible, and where the burden of disease can be considerably reduced using such approaches. Because of the dramatic forms of interventional therapy available to those with breast cancer genes, this is unlikely, in the UK, to be utilised widely. The situation may change, however, should agents such as tamoxifen be shown to be therapeutic with benefits in individuals with this predisposition. Similarly, other genetic variants, such as those responsible for haemochromatosis, can be relatively easily screened at present and will provide an opportunity to significantly reduce the morbidity and mortality from this disease, using simple forms of early intervention such as venesection. It is unlikely that all individuals undergoing predictive testing in this substantially expanded arena are likely to enjoy the benefits of genetic counselling. Screening, even for these relatively highly penetrant single gene disorders, is likely to occur outside of clinical genetics units, most probably in the hands of subspecialists interested in the disease itself. The counselling available for individuals entering such genetic testing programmes is likely to be no more than those entering existing non-genetic screening programmes.

Risk factor detection

There are fundamental differences between predictive testing using DNA variants to detect genetic abnormalities that are highly penetrant and can be used to predict, with high degrees of certainty, the risk of disease in an individual, and those DNA variants which provide evidence of risk in populations but are considerably less useful in individual patients. Most of the genes responsible for common disease will be the latter, that is they will account for some of the risk of developing an individual disease but, because of the complex interplay between multiple genetic determinants in the environment, cannot in any way be used as predictive factors in an individual patient. There has been much confusion about this in clinical circles as the concept of genetic testing has been mistakenly transferred from highly penetrant single gene disorders to low penetrance risk factors defined by DNA testing. This has extremely important implications for the management of such testing programmes and, in particular, the ethical considerations involved in such genetic analyses. There is already extensive experience in evaluating risk factors of a variety of kinds in populations. Hypertension or high cholesterol are both examples of important risk factors. Indeed, both these risk factors are probably accounted for substantially by a range of genetic factors and the phenotype that is measured is a culmination of those genetics factors and some environmental determinants. The screening of individuals for such risk factors is now well evaluated and the ethical issues associated with such presymptomatic testing have been widely and carefully considered. There is little or no difference between this form of risk factor detection and that associated with the identification of risk factors at the level of DNA.

The importance of this distinction is that it should be feasible to do large scale analysis of risk factors to provide information and risk stratification across a wide number of diseases as the disease susceptibility genes are increasingly cloned and characterised.

There are already some important examples of susceptibility genes which may in the future be used to predict risk and possibly also aid in early therapy. The best single example is the ApoE 4 allele, an allele at the ApoE locus with a frequency of 15%. This allele has been shown to contribute substantially to the risk of developing Alzheimer's disease in many different studies. Individuals with one ApoE 4 allele are at increased risk of developing Alzheimer's disease. The risk is even greater in those who are ApoE 4 homozygous. Interestingly, new therapies for Alzheimer's disease have been shown to be differentially effective in ApoE 4 positive and negative populations with this clinical syndrome. It is possible therefore that this genetic information may be used to identify people early in the course of disease and possibly also predict those likely to respond to therapy or even particular environmental alterations, such as change in diet.

Applications of genetic testing

As a host of disease susceptibility genes are characterised, testing for these is likely to be commonplace in all forms of clinical medicine. Two different groups of individuals are likely to benefit from such testing. These include presymptomatic patient populations, and those who have been diagnosed as having a particular condition and who need to be most appropriately managed.

Presymptomatic testing

The use of presymptomatic testing will be driven by the availability of therapeutic agents that can be used early in the course of disease for the identification of environmental factors which have a significant effect on disease initiation or progression. Many of these opportunities are likely to arise as genetics permits a more accurate disease definition and, hence, a more precise mechanism for defining disease subtypes and their relevant environmental factors. Early exposure to allergens may prove to be an important factor in susceptibility in asthma and, hence, genetic prediction for those at risk of particular forms of this disease would be of some benefit, even if only used to reduce the allergen exposure. Early interventions already exist for many forms of vascular disease and the availability of genetic susceptibility factors that could be used to identify individuals at high risk can be used in conjunction with the identification of other environmental risk factors, such as smoking, to identify subsets of the population who would benefit from early forms of therapy. In Type 1 diabetes it is clear that the autoimmune process that eventually damages and destroys the pancreatic beta cells begins many years before patients present with the disease. This provides an opportunity to intervene with immunomodulatory therapy at an early stage in this disorder if individuals at high risk of the disease could be identified. It is likely that genetics will play an important part in identifying the subset of the population most likely to benefit from such screening programmes.

Testing in symptomatic patients

The other major application of genetic testing will be in individuals who present with symptoms. In this event, genetics is likely to be used for a wide number of purposes in the diagnosis and management of individuals. First, genetic testing is likely to help establish more accurate diagnoses in such patients by providing insight into particular mechanistic disease subtypes. This will have an important implication for predicting the natural history of the disease, as will the presence of particular disease modifier polymorphisms, or genes responsible for conferring risk of complications in diseases such as diabetes. In this population of patients, decisions about management of patients is likely to be closely allied to genetic information with all aspects of pharmaco-genomic technology being applicable as appropriate therapies are chosen. Information about disease mechanisms may also provide opportunities for environmental variation, which may also prove to be effective therapy for the disease. On balance, therefore, it is likely that genetic testing will provide essential information on almost all parts of the diagnostic and therapeutic process in the future. It is likely to be sufficiently widespread that systematic testing of individuals may provide sets of genetic data which reside as a database for practising clinicians.

Limitations and time lines

Much of what has been discussed in this chapter can be predicted by information which we currently have available. The overall implications of genetics to all aspects of medicine are now inevitable. What is much less certain is over what time these changes are likely to be introduced and what implications this has for the training of health-care professionals and the education of the public at large. The pace at which human genetics is moving is continually accelerating, driven largely by new technologies and large commercial resources. This is likely to mean a rapid development of maps of the genome containing large numbers of single nucleotides and a fairly rapid progression, through linkage and association studies, to the detection of polymorphisms that contribute to disease susceptibility and therapeutic response. The use of genetics for the development of novel therapeutic agents, and the combined use of diagnostics and therapeutics together, is likely to rapidly drive the requirement for genetic testing into the health-care system. This may be further accelerated by demands by drug regulators that new therapeutic agents are used only in particular subtypes of the population that are likely to receive benefit as defined by genetic factors.

Table 2.3   Pharmacogenetic applications – examples

Cancer
Thiopurine *S*-methyltransferase deficiency
Dihydropyrimidine dehydrogenase deficiency
Cyclophosphamide metabolism
Ataxia telangiectasia

Neurological and psychiatric
Apo E and Alzheimer's disease
Anaesthesia
    Succinylcholine sensitivity
    Malignant hyperthermia
Cytochrome P450 effects and psychotropic drugs
Clozapine and 5-HT receptors
Migraine
Drug addiction

Cardiovascular
Debrisoquine
N-acetylation polymorphism: procainamide and hydralazine
Cholesterol ester transfer protein
    Long Q–T syndrome
    Anticoagulation (Factor V, Warfarin)
β adrenoreceptors

Infectious diseases
Identification of pathogens
Drug resistance

Implementation of genetics and health care will, however, require several other factors. Much of the genetic information will need to be tested in large patient cohorts to establish the real contribution of disease susceptibility variants to risk, and to determine the real effects of genes and their interactions with other genes and environment in the population. Additional complexity will come from the study of varying ethnic groups, particularly with the DNA variants being studied are likely to be in linkage disequilibrium with functional variants. As with all new innovations, implementation should rely on solid evidence of benefit.

The following colleagues were invited to act as commentators on early drafts:

Dr Eric Meslin
Executive Director, National Bioethics Advisory Commission, Rockville, Maryland, USA

Professor William Cookson
Wellcome Trust Senior Clinical Research Fellow, Nuffield Depart-

ment of Clinical Medicine, John Radcliffe Hospital, Oxford

Dr Jonathan Flint
Wellcome Trust Senior Clinical Fellow & Honorary Consultant Psychologist, Institute of Molecular Medicine, Headington, Oxford

Professor Diane Cox
Professor of Human Genetics, University of Alberta, Hospital for Sick Children, Toronto, Ontario, Canada

Dr Mark Edwards
Scientific Director, Oxagen, Abingdon, Oxfordshire, UK

3 Engineering

David Delpy

Introduction

The tremendous scientific and technical developments which have occurred in health care over the past 50 years may have increased our understanding of the causes and progression of diseases, but the limitations of our technology have also defined the way in which health is provided. The existing NHS structure with its local GP, district general hospital and specialist teaching hospital was designed to cope with the provision of health care not only to a population with very different demographics (and disease profile) to what we face in the next 50 years, but was also based around health-care technologies as they existed in 1948.

How then will health care be provided over the next 50 years? The one common trend that has come out from most of the published attempts at "crystal ball gazing" is the devolution of provision to a much more local level, with patients only being referred to a smaller number of highly specialist centres for treatment of more complex problems. This can only be made possible by technical developments which enable the provision of much greater diagnostic information at a local level combined with the expertise to understand this data, make correct decisions from it, and having the facilities to implement appropriate therapy.

Improved diagnostic and therapeutic ability at a local level requires the development of new, or the adaptation of existing instrumentation that is simple to use and which is highly reliable. (It should be noted that such developments imply a deskilling of the roles of those professions that previously provided these services.) This trend has already been noticeable over the past 30 years (and increasingly over the last 10) in the provision of diagnostic services in major hospitals, where tests which previously would have been carried out in centralised specialist laboratories are now increasingly being done at the bedside. This trend has been called "POC" (i.e. "point of care") provision, but this only represents a "half-way house", the ideal surely being "PON" (i.e. "point of need") provision, which includes the patients monitoring themselves at home. Associated with these developments will be the necessity for the information being provided to be correct. The costs to the existing health service of repeated tests and treatments (due to a wide variety of causes) is considerable, yet until the increasing scrutiny by private health insurance providers there was surprisingly little protest from health care providers. (Being cynical, one would not have expected much comment from the commercial suppliers of diagnostic and therapeutic equipment because the increased volume of work merely increased profits!) Technological developments in all other aspects of our life mean that we are now surrounded by complex equipment (cars, TVs, Hi-Fi, mobile phones, etc.) that we expect to work correctly first time, every time. Medical equipment in the future will have to be designed with exactly the same expectations – "right first time". This maxim will also apply all the way through the NHS, where increasingly sophisticated (and costly) techniques will be used, but if the end result of these is to get the whole treatment right first time, the overall cost will be lower than at present where significant numbers of patients require repeated treatments over extended periods, often it must be said to correct problems caused either by incorrect or imprecise initial diagnosis and treatment.

Right first time health care requires not only the provision of correct diagnostic information and precise treatment, but also the expertise to understand the information and draw correct conclusions. Providing this expertise at a local level is difficult given the large volume of relevant information, and the relative infrequency with which a particular disease/combination of diseases may be met by the average GP. This will be alleviated to some extent by the trend towards the larger "group practice" or "local health centre", improvements in information technology with easier access to specialists via the internet ("Telemedicine") and increased provision of re-training (again possibly via the internet). However, it is likely that support will increasingly be provided by software programs. These have been given various names over the past 30 years, from "Artificial Intelligences" to the latest "Clinical Decision Support Systems" (the names have generally reflected trends within the research funding agencies). The use of these programs has significant implications for the possible "deskilling" of the role of the clinician that will have to be faced by the profession. In *The*

Hitch-hikers Guide to the Galaxy,[1] the author Douglas Adams describes in disparaging (but highly amusing) tones the artificial intelligences developed by the "Sirius Cybernetics Corporation" which have "GPP" (i.e. Genuine People Personalities – "your plastic pal who's fun to be with"). While highly amusing, this is precisely the aim of research workers in this area, and the rate of progress in voice communication with computers is such that it seems certain that within a decade relatively "normal" conversation with machines will be possible. Experience with the current very limited "question and answer" types of programmes has shown that patients are surprisingly at ease in supplying information for clinical histories etc., and once the public at large are accustomed to speaking with machines (which will come about through routine "voice-type" word-processing, interactive TV and video games, etc.), it is likely that the public at large will accept the idea of an "Intelligent House" that not only assists their everyday business, but also monitors health-related activities. Demographic changes associated with the ageing population, the increasing number of people living alone, the financial pressures to keep older people as independent as possible for as long as possible will also drive the take-up of this type of technology.

Health-care engineering, the subject of this chapter, covers an enormous range of activities, the future possibilities of which cannot adequately be dealt with in this limited space. This chapter therefore consists of a series of short essays highlighting possible (and hopefully realistic) developments in five specific areas which cover everything from specialist provision in major "centres of excellence" to "across the counter" provision for the general public. The chapter then concludes with a final "Science Fiction" section in which a few more speculative developments are suggested.

Assistive technologies for people with disabilities

Introduction

The last decade has seen major changes in societal attitudes towards people with disabilities, which have attained a new level of prominence with the introduction of legislation to end discrimination and create opportunities for people with disabilities to achieve new levels of independence and a better quality of life. In contrast, growth in the sophistication of assistive technologies (AT) over the same timespan has been disproportionately slow. In fact AT is one of the slowest areas supported by the NHS to capitalise on technological advancement, even if hearing aids, prostheses and orthoses are included. Even more important, until recently whole segments of apparently appropriate technologies for NHS provision have been excluded, including powered wheelchairs for outdoor use, and electronic augmentative communication systems. Unlike many developed countries, in the UK ring-fenced disability-related R&D funding is scarce, poorly defined, and is not strategically developed.

The marketplace for AT in the UK is also very weak, as funding for these devices has been centrally orchestrated with low capital cost, low maintenance cost and high durability being the guiding principle rather than functional performance. In terms of budgeting, the depreciation time for these systems is of the order of 15 years, whereas such technologies in our homes or everyday business would be depreciated over a maximum of 5 years. The resulting low profit margins have led to little corporate funding for R&D, and because the end user of the equipment is not the purchaser, the normal market forces generated by the consumer, which encourage innovation, are not present. Disability-related R&D in the UK has therefore been driven by a variety of *ad hoc* mechanisms, and although some advances have been made, few developments are reaching and thriving in the marketplace. Until a more end-user-focused, choice-driven approach can be adopted, the current wastage of interesting ideas and opportunities for independence is likely to continue.

Magnitude and dimensions of disability

Because there are many definitions and interpretations of "disability", reliable data estimating the number of people affected by disabilities is difficult to obtain. Even more elusive are measures of handicap. The newly created National Disability Council, responsible for advising the UK Government on "general issues related to elimination of discrimination against disabled people" does not currently have an estimate of the number of people affected by their definition of "disability". Other sources of information are the Office of Populations Surveys and Census, which reports a figure of 6·5 million people with physical impairments in the UK and 350 000 people who register themselves as "disabled" with the Department of Social Security. Some "rules of thumb" are available from the USA, and several statistics

Table 3.1   Estimates of functional and activity limitation by age: USA

	% of population by age group			
	Under 18	18–44	45–64	65+
Activity Limitation: National Health Interview Survey (1985)[2]	5·1	8·4	23·4	39·6
ICD – Louis Harris (1985)[3]	—	8·2	22·7	28·0
Functional Limitation Survey of Income and Program Participation (1984)[4]	3·7	10·1	31·9	58·7

Notes: Definition of disability differs for each survey. National Health Interview Survey: Unable to carry out major activity: limited in amount or kind of major activity; or limited, but not in major activity. International Centre for Disabled – Louis Harris Survey: Prevented from full participation in work, school or other activities: having a physical disability, seeing, hearing or speaking impairment or considered disabled by others. Survey of Income and Program Participation: For adults: needs assistance with activities of daily living; inability or difficulty in at least one function. For children: having a physical condition that limits the ability to walk, run or play or a mental or emotional condition that limits the ability to learn or do school work.

help to place disability into a numerical social context. Table 3.1 gives some measures of the percentage of the US population who are limited in performing everyday functions and activities broken down into age groups. It is interesting to note the relatively high percentage in the 45–64 age group, a group now growing rapidly as a proportion of the total population. In Table 3.2, expected life with activity limitations is projected. Although the statistic that a child born today might on average spend 13 years of his/her life with an activity limitation crystallises the issue, these figures do not include the elderly who are institutionalised, frequently with limitations attributable to physical and cognitive factors. These people included, life expectancy with activity limitations is likely to be substantially greater.

Table 3.2   Years of expected life with activity limitations due to specified conditions: at birth, at age 65, and at age 75: USA, 1987

Condition	Years at birth	Years at age 65	Years at age 75
All conditions	12·8	6·3	4·6
Mobility limitations	4·7	2·2	1·6
Intellectual impairments	0·9	0·4	0·4
Sensory impairments	1·0	0·6	0·6
Chronic diseases	4·3	2·3	1·6
Other conditions	1·8	0·7	0·5

Calculated from National Centre for Health Statistics, 1990.[5]

Assistive technology and society

"Surely if we can send man to the moon we can get paraplegics walking again!" is a challenge often thrown out to biomedical engineers, but are we sure that this statement does not just reflect the priorities of able-bodied people trying to normalise people's functional abilities? Many people with disabilities say they have more immediate technological needs which also need to be met while "the cure" is being developed. Only recently has the concept of including people with disabilities in the R&D priority-setting process been considered. The concept that we can do a great deal to reduce "handicap", while awaiting developments to remove "disease" or "impairment", is a central tenet in modern rehabilitation medicine. Assistive technologies can provide us with powerful tools for effective reduction of "handicap", but what societal value is attached to them? What do they symbolise? Do assistive technologies stigmatise? Do assistive technologies promote in the eyes of able-bodied people the concept of empowerment and independence, or do their inadequacies feed our sense of pity? Do they work? In the next 20 years is our society going to ask people with disabilities to "wait out there and make do" while the research community works on a cure, or will society provide the resources to remove or climb the barriers? At present we seem just to be sitting on these "fences".

Opportunities for assistive technology development

Universal design

Although engineering design is often opportunistically driven, in a field where market forces are weak or distorted, some strategic participatory planning will help use scarce resources well. A particularly fruitful approach is to adopt, wherever possible, universal design principles. Universal design incorporates features that help to reduce "handicap" when using the device, but also serve able-bodied members of the community more effectively as well, increasing the market for the device substantially and reducing unit costs. Examples include electrically operated doors, lever-type doorknobs, curb cuts (lowering), and volume controls on telephone receivers. Alternatively, significant cost savings for people with disabilities can be effected if an adaptation feature can be bundled into the product. An excellent example is the Accessibility Options feature of Microsoft "Windows" software, which provides features for a wide range of disabled computer users at a minuscule additional cost to all users.

Another approach is to try and encourage overlap between disability areas through modular design. One example is the development of "smart home" technologies, where there is growing interest in incorporating these technologies into homes to facilitate monitoring of elderly people living alone. However the data buses and sensors also have applications of value to quite profoundly disabled people living independently in the community, both to ensure their safety, and to allow them to control their environment electronically. Incorporating such systems into our new housing stock will save the considerable costs associated with retrofitting.

Mobility enhancement systems

The vast majority (>80%) of wheelchair users have very simple needs in getting around the home, or shops with assistance. However for the remaining minority of more ambitious wheelchair ambulators, the current NHS wheelchair technology is inadequate and at least 10 years out of date. Concern is growing that long-term manually propelled wheelchair use can result in serious orthopaedic problems, such as carpal tunnel syndrome and overuse syndrome in the shoulders. Furthermore, inadequate postural support results in progressive spinal deformity, joint contractures and pressure sores. These limitations, plus the difficulties and effort of operating a manual wheelchair mean that NHS wheelchairs are only suitable for either very fit and energetic young people, or older very dependent people. The middle group of users who need to be very mobile, but are unable to perform the heroic feats needed to negotiate our environment, need some creative new solutions. These need to include lightweight and compactness for independent manipulation and storage in cars and transportation systems, low energy cost for propulsion, power assistance for steep inclines, climbing capability for curbs, stairs and escalators, and the means to adjust sitting height and to assume a standing position.

For amputees, better fitting prostheses are needed especially for the older user with peripheral vascular disease whose residual limb is vulnerable to pressure damage. New automated techniques enabling fabrication directly from computer-scanned stump images have enormous potential to simplify and speed up prosthetic socket production and hence drive down costs. There is also an urgent need for improved orthoses, most of which are still heavy and cumbersome, few including energy storing features to augment function, and whose mechanical failure still frustrates many active users. Ultra lightweight power augmentation for orthoses is becoming more feasible (driven by the needs of the portable PC market!), which should bring substantial improvements in function for patients needing assistance in some movements (e.g. transitioning between standing and sitting).

Communication

As previously mentioned, the rapid developments in speech input to computers will indirectly be of great assistance to the disabled who can still speak. However, electronic devices, which allow people who are unable to speak to communicate effectively, are still lacking. Speech synthesisers are increasingly powerful and more realistic, but the communication rates achievable are still orders of magnitude slower than natural speech, and spontaneous conversation is difficult. Although word prediction and character selection strategies have become highly developed, even the most dextrous typist is challenged to keep up with normal speech rates. For the person with multiple physical disabilities functional communication speed is frustratingly slow. There are opportunities for exciting developments. Neural net technologies should help to reduce the number of keystrokes needed to enter a word or phrase and this may well have applications for traditional word-processing packages, helping to spread their development costs. Small, powerful, wearable computers are already emerging, and should offer substantial improvements for augmentative communication design. A particularly exciting development is the research into direct brain–machine interfaces, which although in their infancy, offer great promise for very profoundly disabled people with, for example, brain stem damage, advanced multiple sclerosis or motor neurone disease.

A fundamental first step must however be made. Our society, and our health-care system, currently must recognise that failure to provide a means for verbal communication, albeit using a computer-based system, is denying non-verbal children the opportunity to develop as fully as possible, and for a dying person with motor neurone disease, the opportunity to communicate with their loved ones in the last weeks of life. Neither of these "outcomes" yields readily to structured scientific study; they are basic human needs that we are failing to address.

Recreation

The importance of health promotion for society as a whole is equally important for people with disabilities. In fact the impact of a disability not only makes exercise more difficult, but also more important. Everyday activities that maintain nominal fitness among able-bodied people may not be possible for a disabled person to undertake. Furthermore, medical complications of exercise for people with certain disabilities requires active, knowledgeable involvement of NHS resources, guiding and monitoring recreational activities for disabled people and elderly people.

There are opportunities for fruitful engineering development of exercise systems for people with disabilities which extend from affordable, compact exercisers for the elderly, to complex functional electrical stimulation systems for high-level tetraplegics. Again the challenge will be to limit costs, as the market for specialist exercise equipment for disabled people is small, and the designs more complex than mainstream products.

Summary

There does appear to be a changing climate for people with disabilities who are succeeding in greater numbers to compete as equals in many sectors of society. However, the NHS provider systems where the cultural emphasis is narrowly defined expenditure containment, needs to be replaced. Assistive technology technicians should become principally responsible for the prescription of assistive devices, with appropriate medical oversight. This will ensure that the prescription process is integrated fully with the ongoing rehabilitation programme and community-based support for the person with the disability. Assistive technology should become a basic entitlement. Funding should be managed solely to ensure that expenditures are consistent with established national rather than regional guidelines. Clinicians should be removed from the budgetary management of these services and be required to recommend the most cost beneficial solution for the patient that matches the guidelines. Approval should be automatic where the recommendation matches the guidelines, and simple procedures should be established for consideration of recommendations that deviate from the guidelines in special cases.

With the ability of users to express their preferences, not only do we create an economic climate for innovation but also a less dependent culture for our disabled community. Along with choice comes responsibility and accountability. In the first 50 years the NHS has been unwilling to liberate this market and its consumers. In the next 20 years this will be an important practical and symbolic step to help bring UK statistics for employment of people with disabilities in line with much of Europe, Australasia, and North America.

Sensing, monitoring, implants

Background

The measurement of 150–200 different types of biochemical parameters now constitutes the routine function of any large hospital laboratory. This analytical capability, driven by the growth in our understanding of biochemical changes in illness, has resulted not so much from innovations in analytical biochemical techniques, but rather from well-engineered automation.

Contemporary biochemistry is geared towards the new imperatives of a shorter inpatient stay, GP specialisation, and more aggressive lines of critical care. Data turnaround, furthermore, is on a timescale that is primarily clinician and not laboratory determined. Near patient testing ultimately provides the most flexible means of satisfying the new requirements, but uptake will only be significant if analysis is deskilled to the level of an electronic consumer item, with the analytical effort adding little to that required for venepuncture. Beyond current biochemistry needs it is likely that short-term variations in biochemical parameters as well as their absolute levels will come to be more clearly modelled and linked to pathophysiology. For this, continuous monitoring of selected biochemicals, beginning with the critically ill through to the ambulatory/chronically ill patient, will demand real-time continuous monitoring systems at least for evaluation periods. Such monitoring is recognised as being indispensable to any intelligent biofeedback system (e.g. artificial pancreas, kidney). Closed loop, computer-controlled biofeedback would be powerfully augmented by the development of robust real-time biochemical monitors. As understanding of the genetic pathology underlying disease states develops, diagnostic medicine will require the technical capacity to undertake gene detection and quantitation at greatly increased volume for population screening, targeted screening and diagnostic confirmation, especially as the list of genetic disease states where successful therapeutic intervention is possible (eventually by gene therapy) increases.

The initial "conventional chemistry" use of enzymes and antibodies as biochemical reagents is now giving way to their immobilisation on solid surfaces, partly as a way of conserving these expensive materials, but also to enable the manufacture of simple, disposable "dipstick" tests. The increasing sophistication of immobilisation technologies has led to "biofunctionalised" surfaces which when combined with new microelectronic (silicon microfabrication) and fibreoptic sensing techniques, produce "biosensors" that increasingly satisfy the operational convenience needs of the clinician end-user. These developments, together with others in polymer science (reactive membranes) and molecular biology (engineered proteins), are all set to play a much greater role over the next 20 years in the construction of fully tailored sensing and measurement interfaces.

In vitro sensors and biosensors – the next 20 years

With increasing assay decentralisation coincident with the need for greater assay flexibility, there will be a much greater role for versatile, portable instrumentation; it is here that a quantitative dipstick sensor will come into its own. Unlike a conventional dipstick it is ideally adapted to a direct electrical readout and quantitation with minimal operator input. The essential development over the next 20 years will be a "roll out" of such disposables to ever more sophisticated analysis (hormones, vitamins, trace metals). There is currently no lack of innovative chemistries for sensors, the problem has been the lack of haemocompatibility and selectivity of the associated sensors. The lack of haemocompatibility results in non-specific deposition of proteins and cells over sensing surfaces that masks the real response. The solution to this problem requires the input of polymer and material scientists, and it is likely that a material science that works on one type of sensor will also benefit others. In tandem with this, the creation of better selectively permeable membranes will enhance the signal : interferent ratio, enabling measurement at very low concentrations.

Selective tailoring of enzymes and other proteins for biosensors using genetic engineering techniques will enable specific functional properties to be realised (e.g. thermal stability, binding specificity). Antibody binding, which has exquisite selectivity properties, has been difficult to apply to continuous monitoring sensors because the binding is not easily reversed. However, genetic modification of expressed antibodies, postsynthetic tailoring of the molecule and the use of antibody subcomponents will allow progression towards

53

fully reversible transduction and the use of antibodies for continuous monitoring.

The cell membrane receptor like the antibody has the facility for highly selective, sensitive binding but also a capacity for ready reversibility of this process. The ability to harness receptors in biosensing has been bedevilled by their structural lability. Better structural characterisation and later stabilisation, possibly by incorporation into an artificial lipid layer, should see major progress. Receptor-based sensors have already worked under laboratory conditions, and a 20-year timescale is quite feasible for practical universal receptor-based transducers. The highly ordered and reproducible nature of the lipid layers also provides for quite sophisticated physical measurement techniques to be used to sense for instance changes in fluidity, impedance or ion channel permeability that follow receptor binding, resulting in new types of biochemical transducers which approximate more closely to natural cell membrane processes (i.e. truly "biomimetic" devices). Once again, the challenge will not be of chemistry, but of materials science and engineering.

The microfabrication of devices lends considerable structural diversity to sensors; multiple arrays can be built up, complex reagent and sample stream channels geometries can be created (a form of fluidic wiring), and operationally even quite conventional chemistries could be geometrically realigned and operated as if they were direct reading sensors. This TAS (Total Analytical Solutions) approach is currently under intense investigation. A critical analytical target is nucleic acid analysis, and significant advances have been made in the creation of high-density arrays to probe for specific nucleotide sequences.[6] Further development of these will take place with greater miniaturisation and higher density arrays enabling comprehensive nucleotide screening on very low volume samples. Nanofabrication strategies will be incorporated into these microstructured chips, for example to give predictable orientation of the surface bioreagent layers and to enhance surface activity. The spatial resolution of future photopolymerisation methods used for such surface bioreagent molecules may ultimately allow for micron distance spacing of sensors.

In vivo sensors and biosensors – the next 20 years

Real-time *in vivo* monitoring has been an agreed goal in sensor research for over 10 years, but as with *in vitro* devices, its realisation awaits better biomaterials. Nevertheless, it is unlikely, however "safe" a material becomes, that intravascular sensors will survive turbulence induced surface fouling of devices, so for this and for safety reasons, tissue implantation will remain the chosen site for *in vivo* monitoring. The current problems of tissue rejection and an uncertain tissue biochemistry are gradually being overcome[7] and it is likely that within the next 20 years, clinically meaningful monitoring of metabolites will be possible. There will be routine monitoring of glucose in diabetics, of lactic acid in the shocked patient and of nitric oxide and oxygen for a variety of situations (hypoxia, anaesthesia, shock wound healing, plastic surgery etc.). In all these areas, non-invasive monitoring will become important, but it is hard to see a universal clinical deployment for anything other than cheap biochemical sensors. There will however be a shift towards the use of optical sensing with developments in fibreoptics, light emitters, and detectors (driven by non-medical products). Short-term monitoring (days) will give way to long-term monitoring (months), the latter being achieved by means of partially implanted devices with external connectors, as is already the case with chronic neurostimulation electrodes. A stringent long-term materials stability will be demanded (and achieved), and this may require surface membrane doping with bioactive molecules or by some independent, localised microdelivery system[8] for the ongoing active management of the local tissue response. Short, intensive periods of monitoring in critical care will be based on batteries of extracorporeal electrodes enabling multiple simultaneous monitoring, the resulting data being interpreted by improved clinical decision support software.

Nanotechnology, membranes, bioartificial organs – the next 20 years

A foreign surface, whether as part of a membrane in a sensor or an implanted prosthesis profoundly influences the surrounding tissue. Engineering of these surfaces has lagged behind efforts to produce the required bulk properties because the relevant level of engineering demanded is of the surface nanostructures. Current generalisations about the biological effects of surface charge density, hydrophobicity, molecular mobility and crystallinity are anecdotal or semiquantitative at best. There will, therefore, be much finer tuning and characterisation of interface structures and of the subsequent bioresponse to these. From detailed attention to nano-architectures, more general principles of material interface design will emerge and these will be augmented by microstructures within implant materials to allow the local delivery of drugs or tissue manipulating agents. New types of composites capable of surface regeneration and renewal via bulk replenishment will emerge.

Medical imaging and conformal radiotherapy

Medical imaging: predicted development

The developments of medical imaging and radiotherapy have been major themes in cancer diagnosis, treatment and follow-up in the past 15 years.[9] In 1980 the only 3D medical imaging modality widely available commercially was X-ray computed tomography (CT), born of long gestation, but which rapidly achieved the status of the most important radiological landmark since the discovery of the X-ray. In the 1980s, magnetic resonance imaging (MRI) and spectroscopy and functional emission computed tomography (ECT) (single photon emission tomography (SPECT) and positron emission tomography (PET)) joined the armamentarium of methods to make 3D images of anatomy and disease. The next 10–20 years will see further developments in high-resolution, high-sensitivity, ultrafast image generation as new detectors are developed, new methods of quantitative image reconstruction are found and rapid display technology evolves. However, the availability of more 3D images raises more clinical questions. It will be important to determine how to better interpret the images. They must be registered and overlaid. The spatial extent of functional disease may not be the same as anatomically evident disease. Choices will have to be made of the volumes of tissue to treat by radiation therapy accounting for those to avoid.

Medical imaging: challenges for the NHS

The development of the physical basis of medical imaging has not been matched by equal attention to its clinical implementation. The following is a list (in no particular order) of tasks that must be addressed and of challenges to the NHS:

1. Image registration is bedevilled by trivial stumbling blocks such as the diversity of image format. Manufacturers should adopt a common format and simplify their detailed industry standards. It would help if the NHS purchasing policy stipulated compliance with data standards before purchases were approved.

2. Telemedicine has received popular media coverage and, while it is impressive that simple ultrasound images in one part of the country can be viewed by an expert at another, rapid effective networking of 3D registered multimodality medical images should be established both at local-area level, nationally and possibly internationally. Different NHS Trust professionals inevitably inhabit particular Trust geography and medical doctors will not effectively use images unless these arrive at their usual place of work. Picture archiving, communication and display are flourishing fields but require simplification and adapting to inexpensive and widely available display technology.

3. It is likely that relatively simple 2D medical imaging will be made available in GP surgeries, but this will require increased training in its use and may have undesirable consequences. For instance, it may prevent referrals to specialist centres where, because of the higher workload, there is more expertise.

4. In the next 10–20 years it is unlikely that a geographical balance of availability of expensive imaging equipment will be established. With the exception of X-ray CT, we presently concentrate expertise in "centres of excellence". These centres make valid cases for their large expert staff-complement to maintain, develop and clinically implement such equipment. At present this is the only option but it discriminates against those patients who cannot travel, because of their illness, or will not travel, or are not referred to such centres. It does not encourage geographically remote GPs and trusts to gain new expertise. It tends to propagate the status quo. Yet to widely disseminate access to such vital image information requires the inevitable injection of resources, not just to purchase "scanners" by "rattling tins", but by a conscious programme of developing expert staff established at the appropriate level. Imaging is strongly rooted in physics and engineering and these professional scientists require support as well as that afforded to radiographers and medical doctors.

Conformal radiotherapy: predicted development

While drug development plays an expensive and important role in the treatment of some cancers, it is estimated that, when 2% of patients are cured by drugs, some 30% are cured by a combination of surgery and radiotherapy. Radiotherapy may be the "sticking plaster of cancer" but for the foreseeable future it is here to stay. The development of 3D conformal radiotherapy (CFRT), in which the high radiation dose volume matches the target volume and avoids normal tissues, has been a major theme of improving the physical basis of radiotherapy.[10] As with medical imaging, its development requires the professional activity of physicists and engineers. One or two UK centres have a research portfolio matching the very best US centres; indeed much CFRT research is unique to the UK. In the next 10 years it will be possible to automatically geometrically shape radiation fields, modulate the intensity of such radiation under computer control, verify that radiotherapy is being accurately delivered, predict the clinical outcome via biological models and, if not eliminate uncertainties, quantify them. It may be possible to customise radiotherapy to the individual radiosensitivity of individual patients. Robotic radiotherapy is in its infancy but deserves more attention. It may solve the problem of accurately irradiating the moving patient and moving target. Since "missing the tumour" is the most serious possible CFRT mistake, CFRT is "driven" by 3D multimodality medical imaging. It is thus evident that, given that 3D CFRT is the only way to improve the dose-based estimate of tumour control probability, a centre of excellence in 3D CFRT must have either the same level of capability in medical imaging or at least have telematic access to registered 3D images.

The role of ultrasound has to date been more diagnostic than therapeutic but may in future not only provide a means to monitor tumour regression but also, more importantly, monitor target position in multiple radiotherapy treatments. The daily alignment of the high-dose volume with the target, by ultrasound guidance, has been achieved in a research setting, but requires translating to the clinic. This may provide the solution to the ultimate doubts expressed by the critics of CFRT that while the weapon is excellent, it may not hit the entire moving target.

Conformal radiotherapy: challenges for the NHS

The challenges for the NHS to clinically implement CFRT are evident and similar to those for medical imaging. 3D CFRT is sadly at present largely a research tool. There are one or two national trials of very limited approaches with conventional equipment. There is no supported programme of "transitional research", which will bring techniques, well understood by physicists, into the clinic. Moreover, there is very little support for clinical trials of CFRT. What there is comes from research councils and industry, not the NHS. Indeed the methods of 3D CFRT have been described as too unstable a technology for NHS assessment. We believe this view is erroneous and, moreover, dangerously ignores international opinion. It leaves radiotherapy in the UK where it presently is, failing to achieve even local control for 30% of patients. While linacs (linear accelerator radiation sources) are widely available, the specialist equipment for CFRT is not. As with medical imaging, questions arise of geographical equality of opportunity. We believe that a limited goal for the next 10 years must be to first establish one or two clinical centres of excellence for CFRT, with little possibility of wider dissemination within this timescale. With techniques, which are most definitely not "off the shelf", the requirement for long-term support of professional staff to maintain and grow further expertise is of paramount importance. As Trusts establish internet sites, GPs (and patients) will become increasingly aware of competing options. The educated, net-literate, patient will increasingly demand access to higher quality diagnosis and treatment, and will vote with his/her feet (and money) over where and when they are treated.

Medical robotics

Background

Robots for surgery and other medical interventions are a recent development, mainly within the last decade. A "robot" for these purposes has had a multiplicity of definitions. Essentially, a medical robot can be regarded as a programmable powered manipulator that can carry tools and move them with preplanned motions and forces to execute surgery, therapy (such as robotic radiotherapy), or diagnostics (such as the use of telemedicine force sensors for breast cancer). These motions may be autonomous, as with active robots,[11] or require the direct intervention of the surgeon, as with synergistic robots.[12]

The related area of computer assisted surgery (CAS) uses tracking systems or "localisers" (usually camera based) to give a computer display of the location of tools relative to some target "tissue". The patient tissue is usually pre-operatively imaged and modelled in the computer, although intraoperative imaging such as ultrasound or MRI may also be used. The benefit of robotics over CAS is that the robot can provide a physical constraint to the tool's motions, ensuring the safety of protected regions and the accuracy of cutting motions. Like CAS, a robot needs to "know" the location of the target tissue accurately at all times, otherwise the inherent accuracy of the robot is of little benefit. In CAS, the surgeon interprets the computer display of tool and target locations and makes tool motions appropriately. However, unlike robotic surgery, should the surgeon make an incorrect motion or simply "twitch", no external constraint will prevent him. Thus the surgery robot can provide constrained motions, very accurate cuts (e.g. an inclined 3D plane on the femur for mounting a knee prosthesis), repetitive motions without tiring, and endoscopic (minimal access) procedures without losing tissue registration.

Future developments

Research into Robotics systems has developed rapidly in the last few years[13] and although very few commercial systems are currently available, it is likely that these research robots will be consolidated into commercial systems within 10 years. The cost, technical complexity and difficulty of use will likely limit their placement to regional centres of excellence. Medical robots will require some specialist facilities within the operating room. For soft tissue surgery, some form of intraoperative imaging, most probably 3D ultrasound or MRI, will be required in the operating room. The specialist operating room will have such features as a strengthened ceiling from which to hang robots (keeping the floor area clear), and especially strengthened operating tables onto which smaller items of equipment can be directly mounted and registered to the patient. Within the next decade, standards for medical robot safety should also be available enabling more manufacturers of industrial robots to agree to modify them to be safe for surgical tasks. However, the complexity of the tasks will probably require companies to provide "turn-key" integrated systems for specific procedures, rather than allow hospitals to develop their own system based on acquiring a surgical robot. Thus the robot will likely be integrated together with a preoperative 3D imaging, modelling and planning system. Intraoperative registration of the robot and of the patient to the preoperative models will likely use anatomical features, identified at each stage using a combination of intra-operative points matched to preoperative surface features.

In addition to modifications to standard industrial robots for surgery (only two companies have systems marketed at this time), the development of special-purpose robots specific to a surgical task will also continue. These will likely be mounted on some type of standard coarse positioning system (fitted with encoders but not motorised) that can locate the powered robot in the desired region and then be locked in place. This will permit the use of small, low-cost, low-force robots just sufficient for the required task. The special-purpose nature of such systems, coupled with mechanical constraints, will further simplify and enhance the achievement of safety. The current concerns about robot safety will gradually be overcome by acceptance of international safety guidelines, and accumulated clinical experience.

The lower cost and more ready availability of accurate and fast localisers (probably camera based) will allow the expansion of computer assisted surgery (CAS) to overlap with robotic techniques. This will also allow the independent checking of tool positions to further enhance safety and accuracy of robotics procedures. (Camera developments from the home and entertainment areas will benefit surgery by reducing costs and enabling the use of multiple cameras to avoid current problems of obscuring targets.)

Benefits

The benefits to be obtained from the use of robots in surgery will be in the high quality, consistent outcomes which can result from the ability of a robot to give repetitive motions with an accuracy of position and force that are beyond the capabilities of a human. The ability of the robot to be used in endoscopic, minimally invasive procedures without losing track of its orientation and position will also be of benefit in extending the range of endoscopic procedures. The addition to the endoscopic tip of small disposable force and pressure sensors, together possibly with miniature sterilisable ultrasound probes, will enable high-quality consistent surgery. This consistent surgery, irrespective of patient or surgeon activity, will allow objective evaluation not only of surgical procedures, but also of the devices customarily used. Thus the efficacies in performance of say a particular hip implant will not be masked by a high variability in the cavity shape or position. Savings in overall time for a procedure are unlikely, because quicker cutting times will be associated with longer set-up times. However by helping to get procedures "right first time", overall savings can be made, for instance in such areas as orthopaedic surgery, where a longer prosthesis life will result in fewer revisions being required.

The use of master/slave telemanipulators should allow increased precision in microsurgery, whereby gross motions of the master will result in refined force and position motions of the slave. The forces "felt" by the slave will, in turn, be fed back amplified to the surgeon at the master. The use of telesurgery for surgery at a distance, for example over a satellite link, is unlikely within the next decade. This is because our capabilities in achieving an adequate sense of "touch" are still rather crude and little understood. Manipulation is currently restricted to relatively simple force and pressure sensing, and an understanding of what information comprises, for instance, a full sense of touch in soft tissue surgery is a long way off. Telemanipulation for diagnosis over a long distance will, however, be more commonplace and useful, and the use of master/slave systems in training systems for a range of surgical procedures will be commonplace, as will all CAS training systems.

The costs/benefits of robotic and telemanipulator systems will however be judged not against conventional surgical procedures, but against the lower cost, simpler alternatives of CAS systems in which the surgeon will be seen to be more immediately in charge of the procedure. It may well be that the uptake in robotic systems versus CAS procedures will depend upon such psychological considerations, rather than on more technical issues.

Biomaterials and medical devices

Introduction

Biomaterials have been used in medical devices for the majority of the twentieth century. Although there has been an obvious increase in sophistication and quality of these materials over this period, their evolution has been largely one of incremental improvements rather than major technological or scientific advance for much of this time. However, during the last decade there has been a revolution in the approach to the concepts of implantable medical devices and the requirements of biomaterials and it is this revolution that will control the destiny of biomaterials and medical devices at the beginning of the new millennium.

The old approach

To place this discussion in perspective, we should consider some of the major types of medical device that are used clinically at the end of the 1990s. The story has to start with total joint replacements, where hip joints represent the public perception of the engineering solution to disease. Invented some 30 years ago, these devices typically consist of some very traditional engineering materials, such as a combination of an alloy with polyethylene for the articulating surfaces, or possibly a ceramic-coated titanium alloy also coupled with polyethylene. It is a salutary lesson to note that the original design attributed to Charnley still achieves good success today, typically with 90% survival at 10 years, 70% at 20 years and 50% at 30 years, provided the quality of the surgical technique is optimal. The objective of these devices has been very simple, involving the removal of bone and cartilage from the two surfaces of the joint once the degenerative osteoarthritic changes have progressed far enough, and their replacement with synthetic materials which provide a low coefficient of friction, an extremely low wear rate and a combination of maximum inertness and minimal irritation. Because all synthetic materials exhibit wear in this situation, and as all materials, especially their wear debris, cause irritation, and no material is inert in the aggressive environment of the body, we cannot expect perfection with these devices and there is an inherent limitation to their performance. However, very little has changed over the last 30 years in terms of concepts and principles, or indeed in the type of materials we use, and today the performance may not be much better than that obtained by Charnley all those years ago.

In cardiovascular surgery, two major applications of biomaterials have existed for as long as the hip replacement. Within the vascular system itself there is a need, and indeed an increasing need, to treat arteries affected by atherosclerosis. Again the principle has been to wait until the disease has progressed to such a point where symptoms are life threatening, and then to remove and replace the diseased section with a biomaterial, or to circumvent it with a bypass. Arterial replacement was first achieved in the 1960s. The materials have been refined a little, and surgical techniques may have improved, but the devices still look roughly the same, they operate on the same principles, and they are still confined to the replacement of medium to large size vessels, with no success in the smaller coronary arteries.

In the heart itself, valves, especially aortic and mitral, suffer from a number of diseases, which adversely affect blood flow such that treatment has to involve the removal of the diseased structure and its replacement with an engineering device. Heart valves were also introduced in the 1960s and, although the mechanical valves have now been complemented by bioprosthetic valves, designs have only been marginally changed over this time. The most widely used mechanical valve today was first developed and tested in the early 1970s. Mechanical valves are based on simple engineering principles and the material requirements are again inertness and lack of irritation or, in this case resistance to thrombus formation, and appropriate mechanical properties. The fact that no synthetic material is sufficiently resistant to thrombogenesis such that patients still have to be anticoagulated and the fact that the alternative bioprosthetic valves do not normally last more than 10 years because of calcification and structural degeneration, serve as important reminders that traditional thinking and traditional concepts have severe limitations.

The same type of story, and the same limitations, may be seen with many types of implanted device involving biomaterials. There are, of course, some very successful areas. Intraocular lenses are highly successful in the treatment of cataracts and dental implants now provide a very effective alternative for the replacement of missing teeth. At the other extreme, there are areas where even limited success has been hard to achieve, such as the use of biomaterials and implantable devices to treat the extensive problems of urinary incontinence. Whatever the medical discipline, however, and whatever the precise objectives, the results of using today's traditional biomaterials based on the old approach of assuming that materials have to be inert and, in consequence, have to be ignored by the tissues of the body, have inherent limitations. The performance of existing devices will not be improved, and the range of clinical applications for traditionally engineered devices will not be extended, until there is a change to the underlying concepts.

The new concepts

If the selection of biomaterials for medical devices cannot exclusively be made on the basis of inertness, and if it is intended that such materials should interact with, rather than be ignored by, the tissues of the body, it is natural to ask the question of how this can be achieved in the context of safe and effective performance. What types of materials are involved and what mechanisms of interaction are being considered? After all, for decades the whole concept of the biocompatibility of biomaterials was predicated on inertness and some success has been achieved, so how can we reverse this approach and produce better success?

If we start with the hip replacement model discussed above, one of the reasons why existing devices fail, and indeed the major reason, is that the prostheses become loose. Conventional devices rely upon a volume of bone cement to hold them in place, but this retention is purely mechanical. Devices eventually become loose because there is no adhesion and because the bone responds to the presence of the foreign material (which is meant to be inert but in reality is not) by slowly undergoing resorption. The one approach to this problem which has had limited success involves the use of surfaces on the prostheses which are designed not to be biologically inert but biologically active, or "bioactive". In the absence of cement, the process of interaction of the bioactive surface (usually obtained by a layer of hydroxyapatite on the metal) with the bone is intended to produce a situation of bonding at the interface. This is an example of how the concept of positive interaction rather than negative inertness can lead to alternative methods of functionality of a device. In practice it has to be said that at the present time it is not clear how this approach does perform in the long term, and it has to be recognised that the materials may not be optimal, but this does give an indication of the way forward.

A further example may be seen with the arterial prostheses also mentioned above. The standard type of device has involved a tubular structure composed of a textile, principally Dacron or the porous PTFE GoreTex. In both cases the microarchitecture of the arterial prostheses is intended to allow blood to pass into the porosity where it quickly clots, the resulting reorganisation of the clot leaving a tissue layer on the inner lumen of the device that is in contact with the circulating blood. This surface is essentially non-thrombogenic. The replacement vessel only remains patent in the medium to large size prostheses, however, because this tissue layer is not necessarily stable. This is because the materials are essentially biologically inert as far as blood components are concerned and the development of the inner tissue layer is non-specific. In practice this layer usually consists of compacted fibrin, and in small diameter vessels the geometry and haemodynamics tend to cause the layer to continue to proliferate, thereby eventually causing blockage. The materials for these prostheses have been chosen for their chemical inertness (although even then the Dacron has been shown to be eventually degradable) and their composition has no influence at all on the biological processes. Current developments in this area involve the modification of the surfaces of these materials to actively promote the formation of the most appropriate type of tissue layer, which is able to give long-term biological stability while retaining good mechanical function.

Biologically active biomaterials and tissue engineering

These simple examples provide an indication of the way forward with the new generation of medical devices. There is a great deal more to this revolution than extending performance in these traditional areas, however, and we must explore the potential of exploiting the biological activity of devices in quite different ways. Let us again return to the treatment of arthritis. It is not intuitively obvious that the best way to treat a painful joint is to remove all affected tissues and replace them with manmade engineering structures. Trends in many areas of treatment are away from radical surgery towards minimally invasive intervention, and indeed towards early intervention when reconstruction involves small lesions, rather than waiting for the lesions to progress, irreversibly, to such a point that they need massive replacement. It is far more logical to detect early lesions in the cartilage before they extend into the underlying bone. In other words, a minor procedure to replace or regenerate a small segment of articular cartilage is infinitely preferable to a massive engineering structure that replaces, in a gross and highly unanatomical way, the whole joint.

Two problems arise with this approach. First there is no manmade material that has properties that remotely resemble those of articular cartilage with respect to friction and wear, so the excision of a fragment of cartilage and its replacement by a small inert synthetic prosthesis is not the answer. Second, cartilage is very reluctant to undergo regeneration; in contrast to skin and bone it needs a great deal of persuasion to undergo regeneration or repair. The solution to this dichotomy is to take a biomaterial, fashion it in the form of a scaffold or matrix and use it to deliver those components that effect that regeneration. As we come to the end of the twentieth century, the approach to arthritis should involve detection of early lesions and the use of a biodegradable matrix which has been cultured with cartilage cells from the patient resulting in new cartilage being laid down *in situ* as the matrix degrades. This is one of the early variations of the theme which has become known as tissue engineering, a rather ironic term as it denotes a move away from the traditional engineering approach to one where the tissue is being persuaded, or engineered, to heal itself.

Once this concept has been accepted and recognised, the possibilities for tissue replacement in the context of the treatment of trauma or disease expand considerably. We are no longer relying upon synthetic materials to replace the tissues. We do not have to try to choose materials which have the functional characteristics of the tissues that they are replacing or augmenting, which is just as well because no manmade material has the properties of skin, nerve, muscle and so on. We get away with this to a limited extent with hard tissues such as bone and tooth, in the areas of orthopaedics and dentistry, simply because here we are only concerned with their gross mechanical properties such as stiffness and ultimate strength. Once we get into the realm of the dominant properties of the tissue, especially but not exclusively those which require dynamic biological performance, then the severe limitations with synthetic biomaterials are seen.

This tissue engineering approach will be most useful where damaged tissues have very limited ability to heal themselves or when the extent of the damage is so great that the normal repair mechanisms need some help. Nerve tissue is used as an example. It is well known that nervous tissue is remarkably reluctant to heal once it has been damaged. It is possible for peripheral nerve to regenerate but it does so reluctantly. Biodegradable nerve guides are able to help in this process, especially if they are able to release some molecular signal, such as a growth factor, to stimulate healing during this phase. In the case of skin, everyone knows that it has remarkable healing powers. When large areas of skin are involved, for example in burns injuries, skin grafts can be used, but even they have their limitations when donor areas are limited. An artificial skin has been proving very interesting here, consisting of a biodegradable matrix, cultured epithelial cells from the patient and a removable protective membrane, the result after a few days being the very effective regeneration of the skin. In the case of bone, again we know it can heal spontaneously but there is a limit to the size of the defect that can do this and there are many situations where bone defects have great difficulty in healing. The solution here appears to involve a combination of a suitable matrix together with a bone-promoting agent. The most successful matrix is likely to be collagenous in nature and interesting developments with the incorporation of bone promoting proteins into this matrix are currently being seen.

This latter example opens the way to the discussion of many other ways in which biomaterials will be seen as important adjuncts to cells in the delivery of molecular signals for inducing the desired response from the tissue. This obviously borders on the area of drug delivery systems which have been under development for some time with respect to controlled release and targeting phenomenon, but has to be seen as quite distinct because here, in this form of tissue engineering, the matrix material or vehicle has to play an active role in the process. The early stages of development, including several of the above examples, are involving relatively traditional biodegradable materials, such as polylactic acid, but materials of even closer biological form will no doubt become more common. Polymers made of hyaluronic acid derivatives, and collagen-based material are already in use here. These structures will be seen as either scaffolds around or in which new tissue regenerates, as encapsulants for the bioactive agents, or as molecular supports. Any situation in which tissue needs an environment in which it can be encouraged to regenerate or redevelop function may be amenable to this approach.

Constraints

The public always has to be ensured of the safety of the products used in health care. Medical devices are no exception and there are increasingly powerful regulatory bodies who have been charged with this responsibility. The basic position with the traditional engineering medical devices is that they should be reliable and safe in that they do the patient no harm, while preferably performing a useful function. This itself is not an easy task and there have been many controversies over the possibilities of toxicity or harmful affects arising from the use of synthetic materials in the body (as with the silicone gels in breast implants and mercury in amalgam fillings) and over the potentially fatal consequences of device malfunction, as with heart valves and pacemakers. While it might seem that more natural materials and devices offer greater security than manmade pieces of metal and plastic, this is not the case. The natural materials, at least at the moment, are largely derived from animal or human origins and all of the issues about infectivity associated with transmissible agents such as viruses and prions are causing immense concerns about public safety in this area. If this concept is to survive, some of these related problems will have to be solved, possibly through the avenues of genetic engineering and recombinant technologies. The possibilities arising from these new principles are clearly immense and the growth of applications of biomaterials and medical devices in the next millennium is heavily dependent on translating these ideas into safe and effective therapies.

Science fiction?

The preceding sections have outlined a range of what we believe to be likely developments in five different fields, based upon extrapolation of existing trends. In this final brief section, a few more speculative developments in each field are identified and discussed.

Assistive technologies

Developments in implantable nerve stimulators, providing a degree of muscle control for quadraplegic or tetraplegic patients, has been mentioned. The possibility of direct stimulation of the brain to bypass or supplement damaged regions is highly likely. In the 1960s and 1970s there were some pioneering attempts to implant stimulators which would provide a degree of replacement of visual or hearing function. With our increased understanding of brain function (and hence where and how to stimulate), coupled to developments in microminiaturisation, such implants are now more feasible. There are already on the market implantable brain stimulators that can help control intractable epilepsy without the need for surgical removal of brain tissue. One obvious area for such implants would be in patients with movement disorders such as cerebral palsy. Associated with the development of such brain stimulators, we can equally imagine the converse, the direct control of external machinery by brain signals. This has been demonstrated in a very simplistic manner for many years in "biofeedback" monitors, and more sophisticated control systems have been developed by the military. A technical development that would greatly facilitate this would be the non-contact monitoring of brain neural activity through the use of very sensitive magnetic field detectors (so called SQUID devices) based upon high temperature superconductors.

Sensing, monitoring, implants

With the development of very simple and reliable "dipstick" types of tests for almost any analyte, it is possible that the patient will completely bypass the conventional healthcare providers, buying test kits "via the Web" from commercial organisations that will also provide diagnostic advice and suggestions for future treatments (and where to go to get them). Recent legal test cases confirming the rights of EU nationals to equal treatment anywhere within the EU, and the recent purchasing by UK Healthcare Trusts of treatment for UK patients at hospitals on mainland Europe could lead to a new "Europe wide" health-care business driven by the patient.

With respect to *in vivo* monitoring, if the problems of long-term stability and biocompatibility are solved, then it is possible to envisage a large percentage of the population having permanent implants which would provide continuous monitoring of the most important physiological parameters. Such a monitor could be read remotely by the "Intelligent House" within which the patient lives, and suitable "expert system" software would provide early warnings of potential problems, perhaps book appointments to see appropriate specialists, or adjust diet through its control of the food ordering/cooking process. It is possible that the take up of such implants could be driven by the gradual move towards private health insurance, the insurance companies providing significant discounts for customers who are monitored and hence more likely to remain fit and healthy through early preventive measures and treatments. A further drive in this direction would result from the significantly increased life expectancy that could arise from our enhanced understanding of the molecular and genetic basis of ageing.

Medical imaging

A possible major innovation in imaging would result from the development of a compact intense X-ray laser. This would enable holographic (i.e. 3D) imaging without the complexities associated with the conventional CT scanner, as well as providing improved tissue contrast and new methods for the monitoring of dynamic changes through the use of interferometric techniques.

A further possible development on the horizon is optical imaging using near infrared light that can penetrate a considerable thickness of body tissue. The major technical problem to be overcome here lies with the computation involved in image reconstruction, because infrared light does not travel in simple straight lines in the tissue, but instead is widely scattered like light in a bottle of milk. However, given developments in computing, allied to the ability of near infrared light to distinguish the absorption arising from different molecules in the body, we may yet see the day when, like Dr McCoy in *Star Trek*, the doctor merely waves a machine with flashing lights over the patient to make an instant diagnosis.

Medical robotics

Science fiction literature is full of stories about future worlds in which molecular-sized machines (nanorobots) inside the body can repair damaged tissue and correct cellular abnormalities. While such machines are currently many decades away (and may be supplanted before they are even developed by molecular treatments and tissue modelling), it is possible to imagine sub-millimetre-sized machines which would enable a much wider range of minimally invasive procedures to be performed with very small endoscopes. (It is probably true that, at present, it is the design of the endoscopic tools that sets the size of the endoscope; the light guides needed for imaging alone now can be less than a millimetre in diameter.)

Biomaterials

The major hope in the biomaterials field lies not in the development of longer lasting and more biocompatible materials, but rather in the development of tissue engineering techniques that will enable new organs or tissues to be grown to replace those at fault. These would be grown from sample cells taken from the patient, avoiding the problems of both rejection and infection that currently plague the field. Such a development is quite possible given the rate of progress in the field, and if so, the use of truly artificial "biomaterials" will be as a "temporary fix" while the new organ or tissue grows to a suitable size. One scenario that has been discussed is the growth of a new organ *in situ*, such that it "piggy backs" the existing (and possibly) failing organ, which could substantially reduce the operation required at the end of the growth period.

Conclusion

It has long been agreed that attempts by so-called experts to "crystal ball gaze" and predict the future, results in the identification of developments that are known to be possible, because they are based upon what we already know, whereas the real developments arise from the things that we do not yet know, and hence are unpredictable. In looking back on this chapter we see that this maxim holds true here. It is likely that the majority of the developments outlined here will come about because we can already see the route to take. We may be incorrect in our judgement of the timescale, but probably not of the final outcome. One could argue that the slightly more speculative "Science Fiction" developments in the final section are less likely to come about within the next 50–100 years. However, it should be remembered that all the surveys of predictions set out in science fiction stories have shown that with the exception of the few "grand ideas" like faster than light space drives and telepathy, science fiction tends to be rather conservative and to underestimate the progress that will occur. Whatever the case, technical developments in medical care will mean that for the foreseeable future, people in the health-care industry will, as the Chinese curse puts it, be living in "interesting times"!

References

1 Adams D. *The Hitch-hikers Guide to the Galaxy*. London: Pan Books, 1979.
2 National Center for Health Statistics. *Current estimates from the National Health Interview Survey, United States 1985*. Vital Health Statistics, Series 10, No. 160, Washington DC: US Government Printing Office, 1986.
3 Louis Harris & Associates Inc. *The ICD survey of disabled Americans: Bringing Disabled Americans into the Mainstream*. New York: International Centre for the Disabled, 1986.
4 Rice DP, LaPlante MP. Chronic illness, disability and increasing longevity. In: Sullivan S, Lewin ME eds *The Economics and Ethics of Long Term Care and Disability*. Washington DC: American Enterprise Institute for Public Policy Research, 1988.
5 National Center for Health Statistics, Vital statistics for the United States, 1987, Vol. 2, Mortality, Part A. Hyattsville, MD: US Public Health Service, 1990.
6 Fodor SP, Read JL, Pirrung MC, Stryer L, Lu AT, Solas D. Light directed spatially addressable parallel chemical synthesis. *Science* 1991; **251**: 767–73.
7 Fraser DM (ed). *Biosensors in the body*. Chichester: Wiley, 1997.
8 Rigby GP, Crump PW, Vadgama P. Stabilized needle electrode system for *in vivo* glucose monitoring based on open flow microperfusion. *Analyst* 1966; **121**; 871–5.
9 Webb S. *The Physics of Medical Imaging*. Bristol: IOP Publishing, 1988.
10 Webb S. *The Physics of Three-dimensional Radiation Therapy: conformal radiotherapy, radiosurgery and treatment planning*. Bristol: IOP Publishing, 1993.
11 Harris SJ, Arambula-Cosio F, Mei Q *et al.*. The Probot – an active robot for prostate resection. *J Med Eng* 1997; **211**: H4, 817–26.
12 Davies BL, Harris SJ, Lin WJ *et al.* Active compoliance in robotic surgery – the use of force control as a dynamic constraint. *J Med Eng* 1997; **211**: H4, 285–92.
13 Taylor RH, Lavallee S, Burdea GC, Mosges R (eds). *Computer Integrated Surgery*. Cambridge, Mass: MIT Press, 1996.

The following colleagues contributed substantial passages which are incorporated in this chapter:

Brian Davies
Professor, Department of Mechanical Engineering, Imperial College London, UK

Martin Fergusson-Pell
Professor, Centre for Disability Research and Innovation, Royal National Orthopaedic Hospital, Middlesex, UK

Panaj Vadgama
Professor, Department of Medicine, Hope Hospital, Manchester, UK

Stephen Webb
Professor, Department of Physics, Institute of Cancer Research, Royal Marsden Hospital, Sutton, Surrey, UK

David Williams
Professor, Institute of Medical and Dental Bioengineering, University of Liverpool, UK

4   Cancer

Karol Sikora

Introduction

The majority of people who develop cancer are over 60 years old. The biggest global demographic change predicted for the next 25 years is a dramatic shift in the number of people over this age. Inevitably this will lead to a rise in cancer incidence (Tables 4.1, 4.2). The UK Government Actuary's Department predicts that the number of people over 65 will have risen from 9.4 million in 1992 to 11.8 million in 2020.[1] The WHO estimates that over the next 25 years there will be over a 100% increase in the number of people over 60 years in 31 countries. Although health education, screening and possibly new prevention strategies could reduce the risks of

Table 4.1   UK predicted cancer incidence

	1995	2020
All cancers	241 000	314 500
Lung	43 000	58 000
Breast	32 500	39 000
Colorectal	32 000	39 000
Stomach	13 000	17 000
Prostate	15 000	22 500

Table 4.2   UK predicted cancer mortality

	1995	2020
All cancers	166 500	222 000
Lung	38 500	52 500
Breast	15 500	19 000
Colorectal	20 000	27 000
Stomach	9 500	13 000
Prostate	10 000	15 500

lung, skin and oropharyngeal neoplasms, the age shift is likely to dwarf all other factors affecting cancer incidence. Cancer is thus becoming a major health problem all over the world. This year more than ten million people will develop the disease. Half will live in countries that between them have less than 5% of the world's cancer treatment resources. By the year 2020 the number of new patients each year will be a frightening 20 million. Developing and implementing a strategy to reduce the untold suffering this will cause is a daunting but urgent challenge to which cancer prevention is the obvious key.

Cancer prevention

The world is a constantly changing place. Cancer care, like airline travel, petrochemicals, and telecommunications, has become a truly international endeavour. It is costly – often way beyond the purchasing power of many countries whose people earn low incomes. There are many misconceptions even among specialists of the relative effectiveness of many interventions. Increasingly sophisticated techniques are becoming available to measure the relative benefits of different approaches. We now have many currencies of suffering: person years of life lost – PYLL; quality adjusted life years – QALY and disability adjusted life years – DALY, all with their protagonists and innate value judgements. But epidemiologists are like voyeurs at a scene of mass destruction. However precise the body count they cannot bring back the lost lives or reduce the suffering caused.

Our track record in the control of infectious diseases is impressive. The eradication of smallpox and the rapid decline in poliomyelitis are public health triumphs of our times on par with John Snow's removal of the Broad Street pump handle in 1854. Better sanitation, education and the extended programme of immunisation, which now reaches 80% of the world's children, have had a great impact on global health. We even seem able to meet new infectious challenges as diverse as AIDS and Ebola fever. Cancer cannot be contained or eradicated in the same way but we will need to place far more emphasis on the role the individual can take, albeit with the support of health-care professionals, in improving their health. Smoking, poor diet, and alcohol account for 68% of the risk factor in cancer in the western world, meaning that with enough education and, crucially, with enough support, individuals can be helped to make an enormous impact on cancer incidence. Indeed our success in other areas of public health has led to increased longevity and thus cancer and other degenerative illnesses have soaring global incidence. The failure of medicine to control cancer and degenerative disease will make imperative a complete revolution in "health creation" through major governmental healthy living initiatives starting in the late 1990s. Indeed our success in other areas of public health has lead to increased longevity and thus cancer's soaring global incidence.

Optimal use of current knowledge could reduce the overall cancer incidence by at least 3 million. Tobacco control is the most urgent need. We need to look for long-term solutions here. The politics of tobacco is a complex conspiratorial web of industrialists, farmers, manufacturers, politicians and the pensions business all looking after their own interests. Reduce cigarette consumption in many countries and the economy simply collapses. Governments are naturally cautious. In democracies they are subject to intense lobbying. In less democratic societies corruption, using the massive profits generated by the industry, usually achieves the desired endpoint. How can we simply stand back and watch western merchants of death so blatantly exploit the young of the developing world, associating images of sex, success and wealth with their lethal wares? With forceful and concerted international action against cigarette promotion we could reduce cancer incidence by 20% by the year 2020.

Dietary modification could result in a further 20% reduction across the board. The problem is refining the educational message and getting it right in different communities. Changing our current high fat, low fibre diet with a low fruit and vegetable intake to a wholefood diet rich in fruits, vegetables, grains, pulses are common themes for cancer prevention. But many features of the modern western diet are now being adapted globally as branded fast food makers seek out new markets. Again political will is necessary to reduce the costs to the public of healthy foods and education and incentives need to be given to schools, factories and public health institutions to help them improve the quality of food and information given to pupils, students, and patients. We now have evidence that those with healthy lifestyles and low meat diets have between 40% and 50% lower cancer mortality.[2] More data will come forward from the European Prospective Investigation into Diet and Cancer (EPIC) study currently in progress. This is a good example where painstaking data and serum collection on 400 000 Europeans could, over the years, provide a vast resource for investigating prospectively the complex interrelationships between diet and cancer. Cancer incidence varies enormously across Europe providing an excellent natural laboratory for such studies. And interventional epidemiology using rigorous controlled studies could produce the evidence that could lead to major changes.

It is likely that current work going on to identify key plant phytochemicals involved in protecting individuals from cancer – namely phytates, protease inhibitors, isoflavinoides and isoflavones, limonene, lycopene, plant phenols, aromatic isothiocyanates, methylated flavones, coumarines, and plant sterols – will progress and that very specific preventive and treatment regimens may develop from improved knowledge about the mechanisms of actions of these substances.

Infection causes around 15% of cancer worldwide and is potentially preventable (Table 4.1). Hepatitis B immunisation in children has significantly reduced the incidence of infection in China, Korea, Egypt, and West Africa. Shortly we will see if it has reduced the incidence of hepatoma, which begins by the third decade of life in endemic regions. The unconfirmed trends are already encouraging. Hepatitis C may also be involved in the production of hepatoma. Cancer of the cervix, the commonest women's cancer in parts of India and Latin America, is clearly associated with certain subtypes of human papillomavirus. Vaccines are now becoming available and entering trial. *Helicobacter pylori* is associated with stomach cancer. Here, without any intervention, there has been a remarkable downward trend in incidence worldwide. Dissecting out the complex factors involved including food storage, preparation and content is a considerable challenge. Other cancer causing infections are Epstein–Barr virus (nasopharyngeal cancer and Burkitt's lymphoma), schistosomiasis (bladder cancer), the liver fluke (a rare type of cancer affecting the bile ducts), the human T-cell leukaemia virus, and the ubiquitous HIV (lymphoma and anal cancer). Although geographically localised, their prevention by lifestyle change and vaccination programmes are realistic short-term goals. A major challenge is to identify, quantitate and reduce the cofactors involved in the link between infection and carcinogenesis. In some examples nearly the whole population carries the infection yet only a proportion will get cancer. Cofactors may have both positive and negative effects, making the analysis difficult.

The key to success in cancer prevention is careful targeting. Clearly there is little point telling the dark-skinned village fishermen of Southern India to avoid sunbathing on the beach. Targeted prevention programmes are very cost effective and can be shared by different countries with similar cancer patterns. Countries with limited resources need not keep reinventing the wheel. Prevention packages can be tailored and adapted widely. To do this we need good data of incidence in relation to geography. Descriptive epidemiology provides a fertile hunting ground for patterns of carcinogenesis. Relating genetic changes in cancer to their cause and geography – the emerging discipline of molecular epidemiology – will complete the circle and point the way to specific interventions.[3] The future of prevention will almost surely be about using such techniques to carefully target preventive strategies to those who would benefit most. In the postgenomic era it is likely that cancer prevention programmes, at least in developed countries, will be completely individualised – a combination of genetic, environmental and lifestyle data will be used to construct very specific personalised messages.[4] One of the biggest problems is education. The media often exaggerate cancer risks, diluting the real public message that is needed.

Screening

Screening for cancer is a potentially important tool. Careful targeting is required – breast cancer is simply not a major problem in many parts of the world. Again the cost of the technology required must match the gain. Low cost direct inspection techniques for oral and cervical cancer by health workers seem attractive to achieve tumour downstaging and hence better survival results. Unfortunately the evaluation of such programmes in India, China and Russia have shown surprisingly poor results in terms of overall effectiveness. A major cost in instituting any screening procedure is simply getting the message to the people and then developing the logistics, often under difficult conditions. Cultural barriers may be insurmountable without better education, especially of girls, who as mothers will become responsible for family health. Low technology tests have low specificity so flooding already hard pressed secondary care facilities with patients with non-life-threatening abnormalities.

Genetic predisposition

Evidence that genetic background can increase the risk of developing cancer comes from three sources. First the risk of

Table 4.3   Rare clinical syndroms associated with increased specific cancer risk

Syndrome	Tumours
Ataxia telangiectasis	Lymphoma, leukaemia
MEN 1	Parathyroid, pancreas, pituitary
MEN 2A	Thyroid, phaeochromocytoma
Familial polyposis coli	Colorectal
Von Hippel-Lindau	Renal cell, angiomas
Neurofibromatosis type 1	Neurofibroma, glioma

cancer is greater amongst family members of patients with cancer. This is currently the most difficult observation to examine mechanistically as the number of genes involved and their functional abnormalities are diverse. Second there are specific families with a very high incidence of particular forms of tumours. Such cancer families may contain mutated specific genes which increase cancer risk through various mechanisms. Some of the genes have been identified such as *TP53* in the Li–Fraumeni syndrome. Finally there are specific recognisable inherited clinical syndromes associated with rare cancer types, such as multiple endocrine neoplasia 1 with its high incidence of parathyroid, endocrine pancreatic and anterior pituitary tumours (Table 4.3). A common feature in all types of familial cancer is its tendency to occur at an earlier age, to be multiple, and to occur bilaterally when paired organs exist.[5]

Until now genetic risk assessment for cancer has been confined to the relatively rare inherited syndromes. This is likely to change dramatically over the next few years.[6] Gene hunting has already uncovered sets of genes which if mutated may result in increased cancer risk. Table 4.4 lists examples of such genes for breast cancer.

The human genome project continues to provide detailed sequencing data.[7] It is estimated that the whole genome will be completed by 2005. Novel assays for DNA mutations which can be

Table 4.4   Genes in which mutations may carry an increased risk of breast cancer

BRCA1
BRCA2
ataxia telangiectasia
TP 53
androgen receptor

rapidly applied to tiny samples of human tissue are being developed. Finally, advances in information technology will lead to more powerful computer storage and retrieval of sequence-based information.[8]

There is considerable public concern at genetic risk assessment. The use of genetic information for life assurance, health insurance and job selection are areas of profound ethical debate. Furthermore, preimplantation diagnosis for known inherited cancer predisposing genes is already possible. As our knowledge of the human genome increases exponentially over the next decade it is likely that selection of low cancer incidence embryos will be feasible. Genetic information will be useful in identifying individually tailored screening programmes, lifestyle advice, and, if necessary, preventive interventions to individuals. The latter may include gene therapy in a prophylactic setting as well as ablative surgery and chemoprevention.

As well as determining the risk of developing cancer, similar technology will be used to assess prognosis and the choice of therapy. The pathway a tumour will envolve is determined by the somatic genetic changes that led to the malignant cell in the first place. "Molecular stamp collecting" and long-term computer analysis will almost certainly revolutionise clinical decision making, especially in choosing how aggressive to be to prevent recurrence.

Surgery

The last two decades have seen an increasing trend to conservation surgery, with organ preservation in several parts of the body. This has been driven by a combination of technological improvements, clinical trials, and patient preference. Thus, breast, rectal, bone, skin and head and neck surgical excisions are now far less extensive and destructive, both physically and psychologically.[9] Molecular analysis of biopsy samples is likely to provide an effective profile of tumour behaviour in an individual patient. Novel imaging techniques will give a better understanding of the anatomical relationships between tumour and normal tissue making the optimal plane of dissection clearer. Computerisation and robotics will allow cancer surgery to be planned in advance and carried out at least in part by non-manually controlled devices further enhancing tissue conservation.[10] The surgeon of the next century will be a highly skilled technician, expert in robotics and computer-driven image reconstruction systems. Like radiologists already, surgeons will work from locations remote from the patient, carrying out highly specialised tasks by remote control.[11]

Virtual reality will combine information from touch during surgical procedures with real-time three-dimensional imaging, especially in those parts of the body such as the brain where tumour resection with minimal normal tissue is the crucial objective. Surgery for metastatic disease will become increasingly successful in selected patients.[12] The precise tailoring of adjuvant systemic therapies, together with immune system resetting, will reduce the recurrence rate in those patients whose primary tumours can be resected. With increasing success in detecting precancerous lesions will come more opportunities for non-surgical interventions and surgery may eventually become a rare treatment modality. Good evaluation strategies for new surgical procedures are essential before routine use is made of them.

Because of the great fear surrounding cancer and the strong desire of medical professionals to move swiftly from diagnosis to treatment, patients currently experience complex demanding and frightening treatments before they have properly adjusted to the diagnosis of cancer, and thought through the implications of their treatments. Patients treated in a state of shock, fear and resistance have markedly less good outcomes from treatment, with greater postoperative complication rates, and it is important that the delivery of more sophisticated care and treatment involves medical teams "bringing the patient with them" in the medical process. This will involve making sure patients are really ready to embark upon their treatment having understood what is happening to them, adjusted to their new situation, been fully involved in treatment decisions and become positively motivated towards the treatment, having had the opportunity to prepare psychologically and physically with the use of counselling, stress reduction techniques, and nutritional improvement. Over-zealous and rushed treatment programmes leave severe psychological scars in cancer patients, which does not need to happen if adequate care, attention and time are given prior to treatment taking place. Time lost in the treatment process in this way is more than compensated for by having the patient prepared, motivated and actively involved in their treatment process.

Radiotherapy

Radiotherapy has a 100-year history. There are essentially two ways in which its effects can be enhanced to eradicate localised cancer. The first is physical – ensuring that the radiation targets the tumour as precisely as possible. The second is biological – utilising information on the differential biological sensitivity of tumour and normal tissue to design an optimal fractionation scheme for radiation delivery.[13]

Physical improvements are likely to be driven by developments in the power of computing. The large amount of mathematical data contained in CT and MRI scans will be used more effectively by new planning systems. Technological developments such as rapidly responsive multileaf collimation will allow the shape of the radiation beam to be changed rapidly and precisely even during treatment delivery, so making conformal therapy the standard practice for all radical radiotherapy treatment plans. Computer technology and robotics will almost certainly take over most of the planning, optimisation, simulation and execution phases of radiation delivery.[14]

A greater understanding in the pathways of DNA repair will make the ability to predict radiation responsiveness a realistic possibility. The functional evaluation of radiation response genes – often discovered in other species – may allow the development of rapid and cheap assays from very limited amounts of tissue. Designer fractionation, optimising the timing of radiation delivery to each patient, will be planned from molecular measurements on tumour and normal fine needle aspirates.

It is likely that complex physical and biological parameters will be used in conjunction with treatment algorithms to draw together multiple data sources so that beam configuration and fractionation schedules can be optimised on an individual basis. The therapist will use virtual reality reconstruction systems to assess progress during treatment by direct observation of tumour shrinkage.

Chemotherapy

The major problem in cancer treatment is undetected metastatic disease at the time of primary therapy. For many of the common tumours our systemic treatments are inadequate and there have been essentially few advances over the last 50 years (Table 4.5). Table 4.6 examines the current status of chemotherapy in patients with a variety of metastatic tumours.

The key problem in the effective treatment of patients with solid tumours is the similarity between tumour and normal cells. Local therapies such as surgery and radiotherapy can succeed, but only if

Table 4.5   Advances in chemotherapy over the last 25 years

Successful cure of some rare tumours
Adjuvant chemotherapy for certain patients with breast, colon, sarcomas and
  childhood tumours
Adjuvant hormone therapy for breast cancer
Hormonal treatment for prostate cancer
High-dose chemotherapy for lymphomas-leukaemias
Effective supportive care during chemotherapy administration
Better organisation of chemotherapy delivery

the malignant cells are confined to the area treated. This is so in around one-third of cancer patients. For the majority, some form of systemic selective therapy is required. While there are many cytotoxic drugs available, only a small proportion of patients are actually cured by their use. The success stories of Hodgkin's disease, non-Hodgkin's lymphoma, childhood leukaemia, chorio-carcinoma and germ cell tumours have just not materialised for the common cancers such as those of the lung, breast or colon.[15] Despite enormous efforts in new drug development, clinical trials of novel drug combinations, the addition of cytokines, high-dose regimens and even bone marrow rescue procedures, the gains in survival have been marginal. Against this disappointing clinical backdrop we have seen an explosion of information on the molecular biology of cancer. Although our knowledge of growth control is still rudimentary, we have at last had the first glimpse of its complexity. This has brought a new vision with which to develop novel selective mechanisms to destroy tumours.[16] This does, however, raise the question over the fact that currently 70% of the cancer budget is being spent in the last 6 months of patients' lives, often on fairly ineffective, expensive chemotherapeutic regimens. A hard but necessary decision will need to be taken to invest more of this money in the earlier phases of the illness in provision of

Table 4.6   Effectiveness of chemotherapy in patients with metastatic cancer

High CR – high cure	High CR – low cure	Low CR – low cure
Acute leukaemia	Ovary	Pancreas
Hodgkin's disease	Breast	Colon
Choriocarcinoma	Small cell lung carcinoma	Non-small cell lung carcinoma
Testicular	Non-Hodgkin's lymphoma	Glioma
Burkitt's lymphoma	Sarcomas	Prostate
Childhood tumours	Head and neck	Stomach

support measures to help strengthen the individual's coping style, and in increasing involvement of patients in the promotion of their own health, well-being, and quality of life. Improvements in mental state and positive involvement in self-help programmes will make it easier for patients to say no to "last ditch" medical interventions, due to their greatly improved quality of life and peace of mind.

The next decade should see a new golden age of drug discovery. This will not be based on empirical screening programmes as in the past, but on logical drug design using molecular graphics to produce novel structures that will interfere with specific biological processes vital for growth. These will include blocking and stimulating therapies for signal transduction pathways; inactivators of oncogene products; the use of high throughput screens to discover small molecules to mimic tumour suppressor genes; transcription control inhibitors for specific genes; selective activators of apoptosis; cell cycle inhibitors and effective antimetastatic drugs.[17] These processes have evolved to use very similar pathways in a wide range of organisms. Thus studying the molecular genetics of a specific functional process in yeast or the worm often will shed light on the human equivalent. The construction of knockout or transgenic animals, where a specific genetic change is artificially created, allows the exploration of that gene's precise function. It is also likely that model systems will be developed to explore the use of direct genetic intervention for the treatment and perhaps even prevention of cancer prior to clinical trials.

Gene therapy

The main problem facing the gene therapist is how to get new genes into every tumour cell. If this cannot be achieved then any malignant cells that remain unaffected will emerge as a resistant clone. Presently we do not have ideal vectors. Despite this drawback, there are already nearly 300 protocols accepted for clinical trial in over 4000 cancer patients worldwide, the majority in the USA. The ethical issues are fairly straightforward with oncology providing some of the highest possible benefit–risk ratios. There are several strategies currently under investigation.

Genetic tagging

The use of a genetic marker to tag tumour cells may help in making decisions on the optimal treatment for an individual patient. The insertion of a foreign marker gene into cells from a tumour biopsy and replacing the marked cells into the patient prior to treatment can provide a sensitive new indicator of minimal residual disease after chemotherapy. The commonest marker is the gene for neomycin phosphotransferase – the neo R gene, an enzyme which metabolises the aminoglycoside antibiotic G418. This gene, when inserted into an appropriate retroviral vector, can be stably incorporated into the host cell's genome. Originally detected by antibiotic resistance, it can now be picked up more sensitively by means of the polymerase chain reaction. In this way as few as one tumour cell among one million normal cells can be identified. This procedure has helped in the design of aggressive chemotherapy protocols in leukaemia and neuroblastoma.[18] It has also proven valuable in elucidating the reasons for relapse after autologous bone marrow or stem cell transplantation where recurrent tumour samples can be examined for tagged genes inserted into donor infusions.

Enhancing tumour immunogenicity

The presence of an immune response to cancer has been recognised for many years. The problem is that human tumours seem to be predominantly weakly immunogenic. If ways could be found to elicit a more powerful immune stimulus, then effective immunotherapy could become a reality. Several observations from murine tumours indicate that one reason for weak immunogenicity of certain tumours is the failure to elicit a T helper cell response. This in turn releases the necessary cytokines to stimulate the production of cytolytic T cells which can destroy tumours. The expression of cytokine genes such as interleukin 2 (IL2), tumour necrosis factor (TNF) and interferon in tumour cells has been shown to bypass the need for T helper cells in mice. Similar clinical experiments are now in progress. Melanoma cells have been prepared from biopsies and infected with retrovirus containing the IL2 gene. These cells are being used as a vaccine to elicit a more powerful immune response.[19]

Vectoring cytokines to tumours

Cytokines such as the interferons and interleukins have been actively explored for their tumoricidal properties. Although there is evidence of cytotoxicity, their side effects are profound which limits the dose that can safely be administered. It is possible to insert cytokine genes into cells that can potentially home in on tumours and so release a high concentration of their protein product locally. TNF genes have been inserted into tumour infiltrating lymphocytes from patients with melanoma and given systemically. These experiments are controversial for two reasons. First, it appears from *in vitro* studies that the amount of TNF expressed from such cells was unlikely to be sufficient to cause a significant cytotoxic effect and, second, the insertion of a foreign gene limits the ability of the lymphocyte to target into tumour masses.[20] Over 20 patients have so far been treated at the US National Cancer Institute and formal publication of the results is eagerly awaited.

Inserting drug-activating genes

The main problem with existing chemotherapy is its lack of selectivity. If drug-activating genes could be inserted which would only be expressed in cancer cells then the administration of an appropriate prodrug could be highly selective. There are now many examples of genes preferentially expressed in tumours. In some cases, their promoters have been isolated and coupled to drug activating enzymes. Examples include alphafetoprotein in hepatoma, prostate-specific antigen in prostate cancer, and c-*erbB2* in breast cancer[21] (Table 4.7).

Such promoters can be coupled to enzymes such as cytosine deaminase or thymidine kinase, thereby producing unique retroviral vectors which are able to infect all cells but can only be expressed in tumour cells. These suicide (or Trojan horse) vectors may not have absolute tumour specificity, but this may not be

Table 4.7   Cloned genes   and their   promoters may be isolated and coupled to drug-activating genes for selective expression in either tumours or non-essential tissues

Selective gene	Tumour
carcinoembryonic antigen	Colorectal cancer, other epithelial tumours
alphafetoprotein	Hepatoma, germ cell tumours
neuron-specific enolase	Small cell lung cancer
prostate-specific antigen	Prostate cancer
thyroglobulin	Thyroid carcinoma
tyrosinase	Melanoma
polymorphic epithelial mucin	Breast cancer
c-*erbB2*	Breast and gastrointestinal
c-*erbB3*	Breast cancer
c-*erbB4*	Breast and gastric cancer
tissue factor	Pancreatic
DD-PCR identified	Many types

essential – it may be possible to perform a genetic prostatectomy or breast ductectomy, so effectively destroying all tumour cells as well as certain normal tissue.

Suppressing oncogene expression

The downregulation of abnormal oncogene expression has been shown to revert the malignant phenotype in a variety of in vitro tumour lines. It is possible to develop *in vivo* systems such as the insertion of genes encoding for complementary (antisense) mRNA to that produced by the oncogene. Such anti-genes specifically switch off the production of the abnormal protein product. Mutant forms of the c-*ras* oncogene are an obvious target for this approach. Up to 75% of human pancreatic cancers contain a mutation in the twelfth amino acid of this protein and reversal of this change in cell lines leads to the restoration of normal growth control. Clearly the major problem is to ensure that every single tumour cell gets infected. Any cell which escapes will have a survival advantage and produce a clone of resistant tumour cells. For this reason it may be that future treatment schedules will require the repetitive administration of vectors in a similar way to fractionated radiotherapy or chemotherapy.

Replacing defective tumour suppressor genes

In cell culture malignant properties can often be reversed by the insertion of normal tumour suppressor genes such as *RB-1*, *TP53*, and *DCC*.[22] Although tumour suppressor genes were often identified in rare tumour types, abnormalities in their expression and function are abundant in common human cancers. As with anti-gene therapy, the difficulty in this approach lies in the delivery of actively expressed vectors to every single tumour cell *in vivo*. Nevertheless clinical experiments are in progress in lung cancer where retroviruses which encode TP53 genes are being administered bronchoscopically. Tumour regressions have been reported.[23] A total of 187 gene therapy protocols for cancer are now active (Table 4.8).

Immunological approaches

The last 10 years have seen dramatic advances in our understanding of how human T lymphocytes recognise and in some situations destroy cancer cells. Major efforts are going into the

Table 4.8   Active cancer gene therapy protocols: January 1998

	USA – Canada (no.)	Europe (no.)
Gene marking	30	9
Immunomodulation	47	22
DNA vaccine	11	3
Drug resistance	10	5
Drug activation	20	14
Anti-oncogene	6	0
Gene replacement	7	2
Total	132	55

development of various types of cancer vaccine using peptide, glycoprotein, antitumour antibody idiotype antigens as well as autologous or allogeneic tumour cell lines.[24] Polynucleotides encoding for various tumour-specific peptides have been claimed to raise a powerful immune response under certain situations.

Recently the successful cloning of cytolytic T cells (CTL) has led to the identification of a series of antigenic peptides degraded from intracellular proteins and ending up in the clefts of major histocompatibility complex (MHC) molecules on the external surface of the cell. Three approaches have been used in their identification. Target cells transfected with cDNA libraries have been used to analyse the specificity of CTL clones. This *genetic* approach was used to identify the MAGE series of melanoma antigens as well as MART, tyrosinase and Melan-A. A *biochemical* strategy has been the separation and characterisation of peptides from purified MHC molecules. A third approach has been the construction and analysis of the response to *synthetic peptides* that bind to MHC class I determinants.[25]

Phase I clinical trials are now in progress using several vaccine strategies (Table 4.9). Most involve direct peptide injection with

Table 4.9   Current cancer vaccines

Autologous cell lines
Allogeneic cell lines
Genetically modified tumour cells
Glycoproteins
Stripped glycoproteins
Peptides
Antitumour antibody idiotypes
Polynucleotides encoding tumour antigens

immunological adjuvant, but enhanced responses may be obtained by using autologous dendritic cells pulsed with peptide antigens. Assays are available to measure the immunological effectiveness of such vaccines so that optimisation can be achieved before moving to larger scale phase II trials aimed at determining efficacy.

Psychosocial care

The quality of psychosocial care currently available to patients is patchy. There is good evidence of variation not only in the skills and technology available in many hospitals, but also in the clinical outcomes.[26] Psychological support, counselling, complementary therapies and genuine dialogue between patient and health-care professionals are not ubiquitous.

The next decade is likely to see an inexorable rise in patient power. This will lead to increased sharing of information about treatments and their impact on the quality of life. Already the internet provides an amazing plethora of essentially uncontrolled information on cancer frequently accessed by computer-literate patients and their families. Society is seeing the deglorification of professionals whether in law, government or medicine. The media will become even more ruthless in dealing with inconsistencies and varied standards currently in use. At the same time traditional support structures, such as organised religion, the family unit, and social services, are declining in their impact. Consumerism will develop in cancer care. Already we can see this with the use of complementary therapies.[27]

Complementary therapies have been widely used by cancer patients for many years. The failure of modern medical science to live up to its expectation to cure the majority of common cancers, together with an increasing self empowerment of those with life-threatening illness, have resulted in a dramatic increase in interest in both complementary and alternative treatments for cancer, as well as holistic self-help approaches.

There is a wide spectrum of belief in complementary medicine. In the past it has been seen by some as a true alternative to orthodox medicine. Surgery, radiotherapy and chemotherapy were regarded as evil – cutting, burning and poisoning. Zealots holding this view did untold damage dissuading people from having potentially helpful treatment. Often these views emanated from charismatic practitioners who were far from holistic – indeed they usually pursued single treatment modalities such as electrical and

Table 4.10   Currently popular complementary therapies used by cancer patients

Psychological	Physical	Pharmacological
Counselling	Massage	Dietary intervention
Psychotherapy	Aromatherapy	Vitamins
Healing	Reflexology	Sharks cartilage
Visualisation	Shiatsu	Naturopathy
Yoga	Acupressure	Chinese medicine
Radionics	Acupuncture	Essiac
Psychic surgery	Osteopathy	Homoeopathy
Art therapy	Chiropractice	Laetrile
Rebirthing		Detoxification
Hypnosis		Immunostimulation

crystal therapies, extreme diets with detoxification or semi-secret organic remedies. At the other end of the spectrum, and equally damaging, was the patronising paternalism of establishment medicine – readily dismissing the potential of complementary medicine to help people. Over the last decade we have seen the two opposing extremes come together to share a middle ground, where by pooling knowledge and understanding, patients can gain immensely. Table 4.10 examines currently used therapies.[28]

The pharmacological therapies are especially popular in the USA where a vast information network has been established initially through specialist book publishers and more recently on the internet. They are much less popular in Britain, although vitamins and homoeopathy are widely utilised. There are considerable difficulties surrounding the use of pharmacologically based therapies in an orthodox clinical setting. It would be illogical not to apply the same scrutiny for, say, sharks cartilage or high-dose vitamin therapy as for any anticancer agent. And yet the beneficial results often claimed are extreme but with only anecdotal evidence. Some practitioners of such treatments may well promise cure from the disease often at considerable expense. The psychological therapies also have extreme variants which may pose considerable dangers to some patients, especially if carried out by inexperienced practitioners. These include the more extreme forms of psychic surgery and rebirthing experiences which can lead to longlasting and damaging psychotic reactions.

Many cancer centres in Britain are developing programmes of supportive care using some of these treatments. Most are avoiding the pharmacological and more extreme psychological and physical therapies. A major problem is the lack of high quality research showing benefit. Most of us believe that complementary therapies are helpful in improving the quality of life of many cancer patients. It may even have a small but measurable effect on disease-free and absolute survival of many different cancer types. The problem is proving it through rigorous and preferably randomised clinical trials. This area of research is extremely challenging. Different levels of patient motivation, together with the problems in assessing quality of life, make things very difficult for the investigator. Indeed the gold standard of the randomised clinical trial may often be an inappropriate tool for this type of research which may need new paradigms for its analysis. It is easy for those involved in purchasing services to use the lack of good conventional data showing benefit as an excuse to turn down applications for funding.

There has now been a tremendous evolution in our understanding of the application of the holistic approach to health and illness, which revolves primarily around involving patients in the promotion of their own health through therapies and self-help techniques which strengthen them in body, mind, and spirit. There is now greater understanding and tolerance of the role of complementary therapies in support and symptom control in cancer, and genuine understanding of the need of some patients to seek more extreme alternative treatments in the face of crushing medical statistics. There has been a great settling down of earlier fears that holistic practitioners and centres were trying in some way to take patients away from their orthodox treatments, or that they were even trying to actively exploit patients, but these fears have largely been allayed through better communication and ongoing mutual educative processes. Sometimes patients and practitioners involved in holistic approaches do place too much emphasis on the potential role the individual may have in the aetiology and treatment of their cancer, and care must be taken to give the right level of weighting to these approaches so that individuals do not become over responsible and self-blame if they do not become well.

The public interest in complementary therapies and self help has spawned a vast information network about conventional as well as complementary therapies. The internet carries a huge amount of unverified cancer information increasingly accessed by patients and families.[29] Clearly if handled correctly, such technologies could become the educational tools of the future. However, it must be realised that at present the use of complementary and self-help approaches gives invaluable tools through which patients' "fighting spirit" can be channelled. There is strong evidence that fighting spirit improves prognosis in cancer[30] and patients do need safe ways of feeling involved in the management and control of their cancer. Therefore, even if there is weak evidence about the benefits of these approaches per se, it is crucial that patients are encouraged and not discouraged from getting involved in measures which will help them to feel in control and actively fighting. It is also clear that patients often get very strong placebo effects from being involved in alternative and complementary therapies, as well as a great deal of tender, loving care. There is also increasing evidence for the role of support and self-help techniques in extending survival as well as purely quality of life.[31,32] The next 25 years will see a great refinement in our understanding of which are the intrinsic beneficial elements of complementary and self-help approaches which have predictable and repeatable clinical benefits in allopathic terms, and which are non-specific benefits which are mediated through the effect on coping style, mental state, and placebo.

Cancer planning

The optimal organisation of cancer treatment services is vital if they are to be most effective. Hub and spoke models are clearly the way forward, modified to accommodate the geographical and economic factors of a particular country. Developing a national cancer plan which anticipates technology moving forward is essential for all countries. WHO has developed a series of guidelines in this area which can be adapted widely.[33] At present less than 40% of United Nations member states have an effective cancer plan. This must include prevention, early detection and education programmes as well as coordinated facilities for disease management.

The services available to people with cancer in Britain have been under intense review over the last 3 years. In the late 1980s it was clear that Britain lagged behind survival statistics for several of the common cancers. At first the data was not considered firm enough – different collection methods, varying pathological classification, and a plethora of staging systems were all confounding factors. However new data such as those produced by the *EUROCARE* study are convincing.[34] Furthermore there is considerable variation in outcome now clearly demonstrable between different hospitals. In 1993, an Expert Advisory Group on Cancer was established to help reshape cancer services in England and Wales. It consisted of 15 members from different backgrounds, its task was to produce a plan to overhaul cancer services.

The framework produced[35] essentially calls for a series of cancer centres as hubs linked to a series of spokes – the cancer units – at general hospitals. The idea is simple. If you have cancer then the quality of care should be the same wherever you present – a sort of oncological Macdonalds. The problem now is its implementation in an increasingly fragmented, competitive and dispirited NHS. There have been many local and regional meetings to set the agenda for change. It is likely that a new pattern of cancer care will be established by the end of the decade.

On a global scale, around 60 of the 191 member states of the United Nations have some form of cancer plan. As the numbers of patients grows with increasing longevity it is vital that coordinated prevention, education, early detection and care plans are drawn up appropriate to the epidemiological distribution of cancer types and the economic background of the country. WHO is assisting counties to do this, in some cases using almost no resources.

Conclusion

It is clear that there is tremendous potential for some very exciting advances in the prevention, diagnosis and treatment of cancer over the next few years. Never before has so much information been available about the disease at a basic level. Getting the best possible treatment to each patient will require concerted and imaginative planning of the structure of the services provided. Such plans will need to be specifically adapted to the geographical, economic and cultural factors; the plans should also be fluid enough to cope with changes in both society and technology. Looking 50 years ahead is difficult. By then the human genome project will be completed with rapid DNA sequence comparisons routinely possible by GPs using arrays of gene chips in their offices. Patients will seize control of their health both for prevention and treatment. The global burden of cancer will start reducing by the year 2015, although the number of new patients will be increasing through the effects of ageing. As we go in to the second half of the next century, cancer will be a relatively rare illness in the developed world, although sadly it will continue to increase in poorer countries.

References

1 *Our vision for cancer.* Imperial Cancer Research Fund, London, 1995.
2 Thorogood M *et al.* Dietary habits and mortality in 11 000 vegetarians and health conscious people: results of a 17-year follow-up study. *Br Med J* 1996; **313**: 775–9.
3 Eeles R, Ponder B, Easton D, Horwich A, eds. *Genetic predisposition to cancer.* Chapman and Hall, London, 1996.
4 Plummer S, Casey G. Are we any closer to genetic testing for common malignancies? *Nature Med* 1996; **2**: 156–8.
5 Ponder BA. Genetics of malignant disease. *Brit Med Bull* 1994; **50**: 517–752.
6 Markham AF, Coletta PL, Robinson PA *et al.* Screening for cancer predisposition. *Eur J Cancer* 1994; **30**: 2015–29.
7 Strachan T. *The human genome.* Bios Scientific, Oxford, 1994.
8 Farzaneh F, Cooper DN. *Functional analysis of the human genome.* Bios Scientific, Oxford, 1995.
9 Gullick W, Handyside A. Preimplantation diagnosis of inherited predisposition to cancer. *Eur J Cancer* 1994; **30**: 2030–2.
10 Brady LW, Mieszkalski G. Cancer cure with organ preservation using radiation therapy. *Frontiers Radiation Ther Oncol* 1993; **27**: 245–9
11 Brown TH, Irving MH. *Introduction to minimal access surgery.* BMJ Publishing, London, 1995.
12 Buckingham RA, Buckingham RO. Robots in operating theatres. *Br Med J* 1995; **311**: 1479–82.
13 Price P, Macmillan T. Radiotherapy in the 21st century; a forward look. In: Tobias JS, Thomas PR, eds. *Current radiation oncology,* 1994, pp. 382–400.
14 Price A. Molecular targets of radiotherapy. In: Lemoine N, Neoptolemos J, Cooke T, eds. *Cancer – a molecular approach.* Blackwell Scientific, Oxford, 1994, pp. 315–34.
15 Sikora K, Price P. *Treatment of cancer.* Chapman and Hall, London, 1995.
16 Varmus H, Weinberg RA. *Genes and the biology of cancer.* Scientific American Library, New York, 1993.
17 Sporn M. The war on cancer. *Lancet* 1996; **347**: 1377–81.
18 Brenner MK, Rill DR, Moen RC *et al.* Gene marking to trace origin of relapse after autologous bone marrow transplantation. *Lancet* 1993; **341**: 85–6.
19 Fearon ER, Pardoll DM, Itaya T *et al.* Interleukin 2 production by tumour cells bypasses the T helper cell function in the generation of an antitumour response. *Science* 1991; **254**: 713–16.
20 Rosenberg SA. Gene therapy for cancer. *JAMA* 1992; **268**: 2416–19.
21 Harris J, Guttierez A, Hurst H, Sikora K, Lemoine N. Gene therapy for cancer using tumour specific drug activation. *Gene Ther* 1994; **1**: 170–7.
22 Baker SJ, Markowitz S, Fearon ER, Willson JK, Vogelstein B. Suppression of human colorectal carcinoma cell growth by wild type p53. *Science* 1990; **249**: 912–15.
23 Roth JA. Retrovirus-mediated wild-type p53 gene transfer to tumors of patients with lung cancer. *Nature Med* 1996; **2**: 985–91.
24 James N, Sikora K. *Clinical immunology, 4th edn.* In: Lachmann P, Peters K, Walport M, eds. Blackwell Scientific Publications, Oxford, 1993, pp 1773–84.
25 Lewis JJ, Houghton AN. Definition of tumour antigens suitable for vaccine construction. *Sem Cancer Biol* 1995; **6**: 321–7.
26 Faulkner A, Maguire P. *Talking to cancer patients and their relatives.* Oxford University Press, Oxford, 1994.
27 Lerner M. *Choices in healing.* MIT Press, Cambridge, 1994.
28 Bell L, Sikora K. Complementary therapies and cancer care. *Comp Ther Nurs Midwif* 1996; **2**: 57–8.
29 Pallen M. The world wide web. *Br Med J* 1995; **311**: 1552–6.

30 Greer *et al.* Psychological response to breast cancer and 15-year outcome. *Lancet* 1990; **i**: 49–50.

31 Fawzy FI, Fawzy NW, Hyun CS *et al.* Malignant melanoma, effects of an early structured psychiatric intervention, coping and affective state on recurrence and survival six years later. *Arch Gen Psychiatr* 1993; **50**: 681–9.

32 Spiegel D. Effect of psychosocial treatment on survival of patients with metastatic breast cancer. *Lancet* 1989; **ii**: 888–91.

33 National Cancer Control Programmes. *Policies and managerial guidelines.* WHO, Geneva, 1995.

34 Berrino F, Sant M, Verdecchia A *et al. Survival of cancer patients in Europe.* IARC Scientific Publications, Lyon, 1995.

35 A policy framework for commissioning cancer services – a report by the expert advisory group on cancer services. Department of Health, London, 1995.

The following colleagues were invited to act as commentators on early drafts:

Rosy Daniel

Medical Director, Bristol Cancer Help Centre, Bristol, UK

Nicholas Lemoine

Professor of Molecular Pathology, Imperial College School of Medicine, Hammersmith Hospital, London, UK

Indraneel Mittra

Surgeon and Scientist, Tata Memorial Hospital, Mumbai, India

Maurice Slevin

Consultant Medical Oncologist, The London Clinic, London, UK

Masaaki Terada

Director, National Cancer Centre Research Institute, Tokyo, Japan

5 Brain function

Leslie Iversen

Brain function and malfunction – the size of the problem

The human brain is one of the pinnacles of evolution, matching in its complexity any other biological structure, capable of amazing feats of computation and memory and in its higher functions responsible for all that is noblest in human achievements and experience. Like any other complex machine, however, the brain is prone to a variety of malfunctions. In Britain about 10% of the population consult their doctors about a neurological symptom in any one year, and if one adds in psychiatric symptoms the figure rises to about 15%. Nervous and mental illnesses account for 10% of hospital inpatient cases, many of them on long-stay psychogeriatric or psychiatric wards.

The commonest neurological symptoms relate to various forms of pain (headache, backache), followed by epilepsy, cerebrovascular disease (transient cerebral ischaemia, stroke and its aftermath), and senile dementia. At any one time in England, with a population in 1996 of 49 million there are about 400 000 elderly patients suffering from one or other form of senile dementia, with Alzheimer's disease the single commonest form, and another 200 000 patients suffering from other disabling neurodegenerative diseases, including Parkinson's disease, multiple sclerosis, Huntington's disease and myasthenia gravis. More than 200 000 patients are recovering from the after effects of stroke and a similar number have recurrent epilepsy

Mental illness is also not uncommon, with a lifetime prevalence of around 1% of the population for schizophrenic illness and 10–20% for depression and anxiety disorders. "Psychopharmaceuticals", the medicines used to treat the symptoms of mental illnesses, are big sellers – they represent around 15% of the total world pharmaceutical market. The antianxiety drug Valium (diazepam) was the best selling prescription drug in the world for more than a decade in the 1960s and 1970s. The antidepressant drug Prozac (fluoxetine) has become one of the biggest selling of all present day prescription medicines, with annual sales in excess of US$2 billion.

The total annual worldwide sales of all psychopharmaceuticals, at around US$30 billion, however, are dwarfed by those of other drugs – legal and illegal – used to affect brain function. A 1996 survey indicated that 30% of British men drank more than the then recommended limit by the government. There are indications that alcohol consumption, fuelled by heavy advertising and unlimited access from 24-hour supermarket shelves, is continuing to increase. Despite various antismoking campaigns some 30% of British men and 28% of women are current cigarette smokers, although there has been a sharp decrease among most groups in the population in the past 30 years in the West (meanwhile cigarette consumption in China and other Asian countries continues to soar). Figures on illegal drug use are harder to come by, but between 2 and 3 million people in Britain are estimated to be regular users of cannabis – the most popular illegal drug. Attitudes to the consumption of illegal psychoactive drugs have changed and are likely to continue to do so as more and more young people refuse to accept government warnings about the dangers of such drugs. The widespread acceptance of the psychostimulant amphetamine derivative "ecstasy" (3,4-dimethylenedioxymethamphetamine) as part of the popular "rave" dance culture in Britain is one such example. Indeed some illicit psychoactive drugs have attained a fashionable, chic status. If one includes alcohol, nicotine and the various illegal psychoactive drugs (cocaine, heroin, amphetamines, ecstasy, cannabis) as a single group of "recreational" CNS drugs, their estimated annual sales worldwide are almost US$1 trillion ($1 000 000 000 000). People seem to have an insatiable desire to alter their present state of consciousness by chemical means.

The latter half of the twentieth century saw great advances in the treatment of mental illnesses by psychopharmaceuticals. The successful drug treatment of many schizophrenic patients permitted governments to adopt a policy of closing most of the long-stay mental hospitals whose custodial function was no longer needed. Progress was less dramatic, however, in the treatment of other brain malfunctions, and in some important areas virtually no effective treatments are yet available. Alzheimer's disease and stroke are two of the most obvious and important examples, each representing a major medical social problem with long-term implications for health service costs and resources.

The following report on how medical research and practice in these fields may develop during the first quarter of the twenty-first century is a purely personal view – as with any other such account the author reserves the right to be proved wrong!

The genetic basis of neuropsychiatric disease

The flood of new knowledge about the human genome that emerged in the last decade of the twentieth century will continue well into the first quarter of the twenty-first century, and from this major new insights into the underlying causes of neurological and mental illnesses are likely to emerge. The idea that some diseases that affect the brain can be inherited has been accepted since the beginning of this century, but these were mainly rare neurological conditions that lead to impaired mental function or gradual degenerative changes in the brain. A variety of conditions that lead to mental retardation fall into this category, and some of these can be ascribed to clearly identified genetic mutations (e.g. phenyl-ketonuria). Other inherited diseases lead to disability that becomes apparent only later in life, as in Huntington's disease, in which sufferers develop progressively worsening uncontrolled movements of the limbs and eventually the whole body as they reach middle age. The disease then follows an inevitably fatal course. Huntington's disease is inherited in a straightforward manner by a single dominant gene – in other words if a single copy of the gene is inherited from either parent the offspring will inevitably develop the disease. Furthermore, the gene involved was identified in the 1980s and has been extensively researched. The gene encodes a protein, huntingtin, of unknown function. Although the disease affects one particular region of the brain, the basal ganglia, the huntingtin gene is expressed in many parts of the brain and elsewhere in the body. The nature of the mutation in this gene is unusual – it involves the insertion of multiple extra copies (between 40 and 100) of the DNA nucleotide sequence CAG, which when translated into protein give rise to a loop of extra glutamine residues in the protein. This change in the protein renders it not merely useless but actively harmful, although why this should be remains unclear. One suggestion is that such glutamine loops might act as "sticky" regions, encouraging the protein to self-aggregate into large complexes, or to bind to other brain proteins leading to a gradual deposit in the brain that ultimately proves toxic. The so-called "triplet repeat" mutation of Huntington's disease has since been identified in another seven rare inherited neurological diseases, so it appears to be a common motif for one form of inherited neurological condition. The lessons learned from research on the genetics of Huntington's disease have important implications for other genetic research in this area. Identifying the gene responsible for a disease does not necessarily offer instant insight into the cause of the disease, nor does it automatically suggest an obvious approach to therapy. Identifying the gene, however, has one immediate consequence – those in families which have a history of the disease can be offered genetic counselling backed up by reliable biochemical tests which indicate whether or not an individual is a gene carrier. Because gene carriers will all inevitably develop this lethal and untreatable disease in middle age, it is not surprising that many individuals at risk have declined the offer of such genetic screening. The progress of genetic research in the field of neuropsychiatric disease will undoubtedly present many other examples of such dilemmas.

Another case in point is Alzheimer's disease. Here great strides have been made in the past decade in identifying a number of different gene mutations that increase the risk of developing the disease. Unlike Huntington's disease, Alzheimer's disease does not in most cases have any clear-cut inheritance. Nevertheless, no less than four different genes, carried on different human chromosomes, are linked to an increased risk of developing the disease. Although some of these genes concern proteins whose function is understood, some do not, as with the huntingtin example. One of the genes involves a lipid carrier protein – apolipoprotein E. This gene exists in three varieties in the human gene pool, E2, E3, and E4. Each of us has a pair of these genes, one from each parent, so various combinations are possible. As E3 is by far the commonest form of the gene, most people carry two copies of E3. However, it is has been found that carrying even one copy of the E4 gene confers an increased risk of developing Alzheimer's disease early in old age. Those who carry two copies of E4 have a very high risk of developing Alzheimer's dementia before they reach the age of 80. Conversely possession of the E2 form of the gene has a protective effect, making it less likely that carriers will develop Alzheimer's disease at all. Some companies in the USA have begun to offer apolipoprotein E genotyping services, so that people can determine which forms they possess. Most professionals, however, have condemned such moves, because knowing the apolipoprotein E genotype has little real predictive value to the individual (e.g., less than half of the E4 gene carriers will live long enough to develop the disease, and those that do develop Alzheimer's may do so at any time between ages 50 and 90). Furthermore, Alzheimer's disease is still largely an untreatable condition. The field of Alzheimer's disease illustrates the likely course of genetics research on other important brain illnesses. There is no simple inheritance and it is likely that multiple genetic risk factors will be identified. The most immediate value of such knowledge, as in the case of Alzheimer's disease, is that knowledge of such multiple risk factors may help us to understand the biochemical basis of the illness, by identifying final common pathways through which the multiple genes exert their influence. This may in turn permit new therapeutic strategies to be developed to target these disease mechanisms.

In psychiatric illness there is undoubtedly a rich field for future genetics research, although the effort has yielded little success so far. The data in Table 5.1 indicate that it is likely that genetic risk factors remain to be discovered for most of the common mental illnesses. Again there is no evidence for simple inheritance – for example, the identical twin of someone who develops schizophrenia has a 50% chance of also becoming schizophrenic, but this is equally likely not to happen.

As in Alzheimer's disease, multiple genetic risk factors will probably be identified for each of the principal mental illnesses. Again this will initially have little diagnostic value, but it may help to provide much needed new insight into the molecular processes that underlie these illnesses – and this in turn may provide new therapeutic strategies which tackle the fundamental brain disorder underlying the illness, rather than merely treating the symptoms of the illness as with current CNS drugs. It is possible that the genotyping of high-risk groups (e.g., first degree relatives of those

Table 5.1 Heritability of psychiatric illnesses

Illness	Morbidity risk (%)	
	Normal population	First-degree relative
Schizophrenia	0.8	6–12
Depression	5–8	13–35
Manic-depressive illness	0.2–0.5	4–9
Anxiety/neurosis	3–6	15

suffering from schizophrenia or manic-depressive illness) could help to identify individuals at high risk of developing the symptoms of mental illness – and that intensive behavioural and pharmacological treatment of such individuals could prevent this happening, particularly when gene therapy becomes a reality.

Other genetic risk factors are likely to be identified that lead not to mental or neurological illness but which confer an increased probability of developing substance abuse or addiction. Thus, it may be possible to identify those at risk of developing alcoholism or drug addiction and perhaps to intervene with behavioural, pharmacological or gene therapy before such behaviour patterns become engrained. Some have even suggested that it may be possible to identify genes that are associated with an increased risk of criminal or aggressive behaviour.

Knowledge of the genetic risk factors underlying mental and neurological illnesses or substance abuse could also in the longer run be used to remove these genes from the human gene pool. Genetic counselling is already an accepted practice, and a new form of genetic selection may become increasingly prevalent in the choice of human embryos to be used for reimplantation, part of the process of *in vitro* fertilisation. These procedures increasingly use genomic screening in their selection of embryos. It is unlikely though that we will follow the Chinese, who do not permit families with a history of schizophrenia or other major mental illness to reproduce.

Repair of the nervous system

The remarkable developments that may be anticipated in the field of brain repair during the first two decades of the twenty-first century will undoubtedly attract much public attention and raise new debates about the allocation of medical resources. Essentially all of the 10 billion or more nerve cells in the adult human brain are already present at birth, although they continue to develop their complex connections with each other for the first 15–20 years of life. Nerve cells which are lost as the result of injury or other events (e.g., stroke) are not readily replaced, although the adult human brain does retain some ability to generate new neural progenitor cells and there is a surprising degree of plasticity in compensating for a loss of function through the rerouting of neural circuitry. However, in such progressive neurodegenerative conditions as Parkinson's, Huntington's or Alzheimer's diseases the cumulative loss of particular groups of nerve cells leads inevitably to a progressive loss of function that cannot be compensated for adequately. Thus patients with Parkinson's disease suffer a progressive loss of dopamine-containing nerve cells which leads to an inability to initiate voluntary movement accompanied by muscular rigidity and tremor; Huntington's disease patients lose nerve cells from the movement control centres in the basal ganglia of brain and suffer uncontrolled movements of the limbs and body; Alzheimer's disease patients develop a generalised loss of nerve cells from the cerebral cortex and exhibit a decline in intellectual faculties, particularly in memory for recent events, making it hard for them to function normally.

Until recently it was thought that such conditions were irreversible as new nerve cells cannot be generated in the adult brain. However, rapid advances in nerve cell transplantation techniques have changed this view. Pioneering work in Sweden and elsewhere in the 1970s and 1980s showed that dopamine-containing nerve cells could be transplanted from rat embryos into the brains of adult rats where they could restore function in animals whose brains had previously been depleted of dopamine cells. CNS neurons only survive such transplantation if taken from embryonic donors and there is a narrow time window in development when the donor cells can be successfully used for transplantation. This critical period corresponds to the time when the nerve cells are undergoing their final cell division and beginning to become committed to development into dopamine nerve cells. At this stage the developing nerve cells are moving into an active phase of growth giving rise to the outgrowth of fibres which seek appropriate targets to connect with in the recipient brain. Transplantation initially used solid fragments of embryo brain, but an improved technique was developed in the 1980s which involved injecting a suspension of dissociated embryonic nerve cells – this had the advantage that injections could be made into multiple sites in the recipient brain and it gave better survival of the donor cells. It was this technique that was used in the first human trials in patients with Parkinson's disease, using dopamine cells obtained from human aborted fetuses. By 1998 more than 200 patients in different centres around the world had received such implants and although the early results were modest there was clear evidence that most patients showed an improvement in their clinical symptoms, demonstrating the validity of this approach. Brain imaging techniques which allowed the progress of the implanted dopamine cells to be monitored showed that some of the implanted nerve cells did survive and they continued to grow and make connections in the patient's brain for periods of a year or more after implantation.

Although these early results were encouraging, the use of neural transplantation remains purely experimental. The use of human fetal material as the source of immature nerve cells for transplantation has many disadvantages: the approach is distasteful to many and unacceptable on religious grounds to others; the availability of fetal material at the most suitable critical period of development is strictly limited; and the cell suspension used for transplantation contains a mixture of nerve cells of many different types, of which the desired dopamine-containing cells formed only a minor part. This problem is likely to be solved in two ways: by the development of genetically engineered animals as suitable donors (xeno-transplantation), and by the use of immortalised human nerve cell progenitors (stem cells).

Xenotransplantation, the transfer of cells or tissues from one species to another, is no longer in the realms of science fiction. The problem with this approach is that the "foreign" transplanted cells are recognised by the recipient's immune system and are then rejected. One way of reducing this rejection response is to use closely related species. The concept of using monkeys as donors for human transplantation, however, is considered unacceptable because most non-human primates are endangered species, and there is felt to be an unacceptable risk of transmission of viral and other diseases from primates to man – after all this is how the AIDS epidemic is believed to have started in Africa. A solution may be to create genetically engineered donor species in which the animal cells are modified deliberately to reduce the risk of rejection. The species likely to be used is the pig, as it is easily available and closely related in body and organ size to man (more important for kidney and heart transplantation than for nerve cells). A number of genetic modifications of pigs are being assessed in various laboratories in Britain and the USA. These include modifying the sugars expressed on the surface of pig cells (a powerful foreign signal to the immune system); engineering pig cells to express inhibitors of the complement system (which is the mechanism whereby donor cells are killed by the immune system during rejection); and combining these approaches with the use of powerful new immunosuppressant drugs. Although the use of pigs as donors for human transplantation raises ethical concerns about the use of animals, and worries about the possibility of introducing pig retroviruses into man, these concerns are probably exaggerated and may be allayed by the dramatic results that could be obtained in the first clinical trials – which will involve the transplantation of genetically engineered pig hearts and later kidneys into terminally ill patients. There is an enormous unmet demand for heart and kidney transplants, and xenotransplantation could create a new industry for the supply of these materials worth many billions of dollars. The same approach is likely to be applied to the neural transplantation field and the use of embryonic dopamine nerve cells obtained from genetically engineered pigs may become commonplace as a treatment for Parkinson's disease by the end of the first decade of the twenty-first century. The clinical improvements will remain modest, but sufficiently impressive to generate a widespread demand from patients and doctors for this operation – with perhaps as many as 50 000 xenotransplants each year for Parkinson's disease, and an increasing number of experimental surgical procedures aiming to apply the same strategy to the treatment of Huntington's disease, epilepsy, multiple sclerosis, and Alzheimer's disease.

The problems of long-term immune system rejection are not likely to be completely solved by the xenotransplantation approach, and the beneficial effects seen in many Parkinsonian patients may fade gradually with time. Fortunately another major step forward will become available in the 2020s with the first widespread use of neural stem cells as neurotransplant material. Stem cells from other organs, for example bone marrow, have already found important medical applications in the treatment of cancer. It has been known since the 1980s that it is possible to obtain tissue cultures of neural stem cells from embryonic animal and human brain. These are the progenitor cells from which all brain tissue – neural as well as non-neural – is derived. However, it has proved technically difficult to find the right conditions to maintain these cells in a growing and dividing state in tissue culture without their converting to nerve cells or non-neural support cells. These difficulties will be solved. It is already possible to maintain stable growing cultures of "immortal" neural stem cells, derived from just a few human fetuses and capable of supplying all the world's needs for transplantation material. It will take longer to understand how to manipulate the tissue culture conditions of these stem cells so that they can be provoked to differentiate as dopamine-containing neurons (or as other forms of nerve cell or support cell). Once these conditions are established (by adding the appropriate cocktail of neural growth factors, cytokines, and nuclear receptor proteins) the way will be open for a new approach to human neurotransplantation, using implants of human immature dopamine cells, but not requiring the use of large amounts of fetal material or the implantation of large numbers of non-dopamine cells. Stem cell neurotransplantation will rapidly overtake xenotransplantation as the method of choice and many new applications of this technology to neurodegenerative disease other than Parkinson's disease will be explored. Implants of nerve cells containing the inhibitory chemical messenger GABA, for example, may be effective in the suppression of epileptic seizures, and the use of basal ganglia cell implants for treating the uncontrolled movements of Huntington's disease could be another major advance.

The ability to replace missing nerve cells does not completely solve the problem of brain repair. Another feature of the mammalian central nervous system is that if long fibre connections are damaged they do not regenerate. This is quite unlike the situation in the peripheral nervous system, where damage to a nerve can lead to temporary paralysis and loss of sensation in a limb, but the nerve fibres will slowly regenerate and function can be restored fully. Even in the central nervous system repair is possible in many vertebrate species. Thus, in fishes and amphibians, for example, damage to the optic nerve may lead to temporary blindness but sight can be restored as the nerve fibres eventually regenerate and become reconnected. In song birds a whole region of the brain involved in the song repertoire is reconstructed each year. The inability of the mammalian central nervous system to repair itself has long been one of the enigmas of neurobiology. Towards the end of the twentieth century the mechanisms are beginning to be understood. The main problem seems to be that in the scar tissue formed at the site of an injury in brain or spinal cord a number of inhibitory proteins are expressed that prevent regenerating nerve fibres from crossing the scar tissue gap. If means could be found to bridge that gap, for example by using pieces of peripheral nerve as "guides", by laying trails of chemical growth factors, or by injecting suspensions of neural stem cells programmed to form helpful support cells, regeneration could take place even over long distances in spinal cord and brain. The first attempts to use purified protein growth factors to promote neural repair proved disappointing, but eventually the right formula will be found for using these powerful chemical promoters of nerve cell growth and survival will be found. Promising results have already been obtained with nerve growth factor (NGF) in the treatment of peripheral nerve damage in diabetes. Another group of chemicals found both in brain and in the immune system, the immunophilins also offer great promise as neuroregenerative agents. It may take another 10–20 years, however, for this technology to be developed for successful clinical use, and the first beneficial results may begin to be seen in the treatment of spinal cord injuries and in the treatment of other forms of paralysis due to damage of CNS tracts. The prospect of making the blind see again and the deaf hear will remain among the elusive but not impossible goals of this field of research. The cost effectiveness of the successful treatment of disabling diseases, allowing patients with spinal injuries to become mobile and self supporting once more, is obvious, but there will no doubt be concerns voiced about the medical costs of implementing any large scale programme of neural repair, particularly because of the accumulated backlog of untreated cases that would have to be dealt with initially and the uncertainty about the long-term outcomes of these new treatments. Nevertheless, the ability to undertake brain repair on even a limited scale will represent one of the most important achievements of twenty-first century neuroscience research.

Comment from Professor SH SNYDER, Department of Neuroscience, Johns Hopkins University School of Medicine, Baltimore, MD, USA:

"In the history of medical science, things that seemed absolutely impossible turn out to be solved very simply and cheaply. Thus, the problem of neural repair may not require transplantation of embryonic tissue but simple drugs."

Stress and the nervous system

According to a recent government survey, around one-third of the adult population in Britain in 1994 reported feeling under "a good bit" or "a great deal" of stress (Table 5.2). This seems to be one of the inescapable facts of modern life. There is, furthermore, an increasing body of medical evidence that stress can cause physical illness, although the link has often been remarkably hard to prove.

One rough and ready way of measuring the degree of stress to which an individual has been exposed is in terms of "life events", each being assigned an arbitrary score according to severity – thus

Table 5.2   Experience of stress (England), 1994

	Experience of stress (%)
Males	
None	26
A little	41
A good bit	18
A great deal	15
Females	
None	24
A little	44
A good bit	17
A great deal	16

[UK Government "Social Trends" 1997 – data refer to all adults over age of 16]

a maximum rating of 100 is assigned to the death of a spouse; divorce is rated 73; marriage 50; changing job 36; moving house 20; Christmas 12, and so on. A composite score can then be calculated. Thousands of studies during the past 30 years have investigated the relationship between life events and health, and by and large the conclusion has been that people who have been exposed to a lot of life events-related stress have a slight but significantly increased risk of illness. Furthermore the illness may be of many different varieties, and people with high life event scores tend to remain ill for longer and to report more severe symptoms.

But not all people react adversely to stressful events. Another popular line of research has sought to correlate illness with personality. Many studies have sought to find a relationship between personality and health. The so-called Type A personality, characterised by hostility, aggressiveness, competitiveness, impatience and outbursts of anger, has been the subject of thousands of studies. The conclusion is that Type A personality has been added to the officially recognised risk factors for coronary heart disease. At the other extreme, the Type C personality, characterised by extreme passivity, suppression of emotions, avoidance of conflict, obedience and stoicism, has been found to be linked to an increased risk of various forms of cancer.

What is the physical explanation for psychosomatic illness? Most scientists now believe that an important key is the link between the brain and the immune system, the body's natural defence mechanisms against illness. The subject of "psychoneuroimmunology" has grown up to study what neural and immune system mechanisms may be involved. While understanding remains rudimentary, it has become clear that the immune system, with its complex families of chemical mediators of inflammation and attack, is reflected also in the brain itself, which uses many of the same chemicals – known as chemokines and cytokines – for signalling between nerve cells. It is also clear that psychosomatic illness does involve changes in immune system function, although exactly how these come about remains unknown.

Stress is also known to activate a variety of hormonal responses, including adrenaline and steroid release and the potent morphine-like chemical beta-endorphin. In boring modern day life – without the thrill of the hunt – more and more people deliberately seek stressful experiences – jumping out of airplanes or off high bridges on a bungee rope, subjecting themselves to frightening rides at theme parks, or the gruelling experience of marathon running. The experience of an acute, predictable stress, followed by the elation of the adrenaline or opiate-induced "high" is one that many seek. It is the stresses of life that are not predictable, or from which there is no escape that seem to be damaging.

We know little about how to translate the new knowledge about the relationship between personality and stress and endocrine and immune system function into new strategies for the treatment of stress-related diseases. One can speculate that this will prove a rich ground for pharmacology in the future. Progress is already being made in devising simple drug molecules that penetrate the brain and block the actions of one of the key hormones involved as a final common pathway in mediating the effects of stress – a peptide known as "corticotropin-releasing factor" (CRF) – and such drugs may prove to be breakthroughs in the chemical management of stress. CRF is present both in the hypothalamus, where it helps to trigger the pituitary/adrenal axis response to stress, and in other areas of the brain, where it mediates behavioural responses to stress. Perhaps complementary to pharmacological interventions will be the development of improved behavioural therapy regimens. It is already known that Type A personalities can be taught to control their anger and impetuousness – and perhaps by exposing Type C personalities to a virtual reality world in which they learn to express emotions and to overcome their passivity they too could be trained.

Drug treatment of nervous system disorders

Dramatic advances were made in the latter half of the twentieth century in the drug treatment of neurological and mental illnesses.

The discovery of effective drugs to alleviate the symptoms of schizophrenia, depression and anxiety radically changed the way in which psychiatrists treated these conditions. Since the major discoveries of these drugs in the 1950s and 1960s, however, further scientific progress has been modest, consisting largely of a refinement of the early psychopharmaceuticals to make them more potent and to remove unwanted side effects.

One problem has been that drug companies tend to stick to known mechanisms of action. One of the consequences is that essentially all of the drugs used to treat schizophrenia work by one mechanism – blockade of receptors in the brain which recognise the neurotransmitter dopamine. Advances in this area have consisted largely of refinements, adding various combinations of additional properties to such molecules to enhance their anti-schizophrenic actions and to reduce their unwanted side effects (e.g., in this case the drugs tend to cause Parkinson's disease-like symptoms because they block dopamine actions). The end of the twentieth century saw the launch of a series of new "atypical" antischizophrenia drugs which combine dopamine blockade with an ability to block brain receptors for another neurotransmitter – serotonin (5-hydroxytryptamine). It is likely that these will become the drugs of choice for the treatment of schizophrenia for many years to come – and further advances in the drug treatment of this disease will rely on the ability of drug company scientists to break out of the antidopamine mould into new mechanisms for anti-psychotic drug action.

Prozac was hailed as the most successful new drug for the treatment of mental illness in recent years – but in reality it too is merely a refinement of the antidepressant drugs first described 40 years earlier. These antidepressants work by blocking the tissue uptake mechanisms which are responsible for terminating the actions of the neurotransmitters noradrenaline and serotonin after their release in the brain. The drugs thus enhance and prolong the actions of these chemical messengers. The first antidepressants acted both on the serotonin and noradrenaline systems, whereas Prozac and related newer drugs target the serotonin system selectively. Such drugs have proved to be equally effective as antidepressants but considerably less toxic – the risk of suicide with the earlier drugs is, for example, removed. As in schizophrenia, what is needed in the development of new antidepressants is a breakthrough into entirely new mechanisms of action. Such a breakthrough may come from the new generation of drugs currently under development in drug companies, which target not the traditional amine neurotransmitters (noradrenaline, dopamine, serotonin and acetylcholine) but the neuropeptide systems in brain. More than 50 different peptides (chains of amino acid residues, ranging from three to 40 amino acid residues in length) exist in different populations of neurons in brain where they act as chemical messengers. In most cases their actions seem to be to modulate the effects of classical neurotransmitters – setting the "gain" rather than acting as "ON" or "OFF" signals. During the past 20 years scientists have learned how to make simple organic drug molecules which act to mimic or to block the actions of the neuropeptides. Unlike the peptides themselves, such drug molecules can readily penetrate the brain from the blood and are absorbed from the gut after being taken by mouth. One series of potentially valuable new antidepressants has emerged from such research.

Drugs which block receptors in the brain from the neuropeptide substance P were reported recently to be as effective as Prozac as antidepressants in early clinical trials.

Comments from Professor SH Snyder:

"You discuss the problem of drug company strategy. I think that this is a fascinating and important issue that has not been adequately appreciated and which can be addressed by governmental bodies. You put some of the blame on drug companies tending to stick to known mechanisms of action. This is certainly true. However, one must place this in the context of the financial pressures on the drug industry imposed by FDA regulations and to a certain extent by drug company philosophy. What gave rise to the big breakthroughs in psychopharmacology in the mid 1950s was the willingness of drug companies and investigators to go immediately into humans with drugs that had some faint suggestion of benefit in animal behavioral studies. Moreover, in these studies investigators spread a wide net, looking at virtually every type of mental disturbance. As you well know, most of the important findings were totally unexpected, hence the crucial role of serendipity, a concept that is important to convey to the audience. The pharmaceutical industry reasoning is that 'it will cost $200 million to develop a drug so we better be damn sure that it will work in advance'. The mistake in this line of reasoning is that moving a drug to early Phase I clinical trials is not particularly expensive even with current FDA regulations."

New pharmacology based around neuropeptides may also be where we may see major new advances in the treatment of pain. Although morphine remains one of the most powerful drugs known for the treatment of severe pain, it does not always work. Around half of terminally ill cancer patients suffer pain from which morphine gives little or no relief. Hope centres on targeting neuropeptide systems, substance P, somatostatin, cholecystokinin, galanin, known to be involved in the transmission of pain messages from peripheral targets in the body into the central nervous system. The first clinical results with new drugs that mimic or block these peptides are expected by the end of the twentieth century, and are likely to provide important new additions to the range of medicines available for the management of pain. Fortunately such advances come at a time when clinicians are increasingly recognising the importance of palliative care – improving the quality of life for the sick and dying.

Another important advance in the treatment of milder forms of pain will come from the introduction of new aspirin-like drugs which target selectively the enzyme cyclo-oxygenase 2. Aspirin and the many related non-steroidal anti-inflammatory drugs act by inhibiting the synthesis of the inflammatory mediators the prostaglandins, but it works equally on two forms of the enzyme responsible for this – COX-1 and COX-2. Selective blockade of COX-2 gives all of the beneficial effects of aspirin – anti-inflammation, pain relief – without some of the dangerous side effects, especially gastric ulcers and bleeding. COX-2 inhibitors look set to be among the "blockbuster" drugs of the early twenty-first century.

The most exciting developments in CNS pharmacology, however, will come in areas where no effective treatments exist today. The past two decades, for example, have seen an upsurge of research directed to the discovery of drug treatments that might lessen the permanent brain damage that occurs after a stroke. In a stroke an artery supplying blood to the brain (often one which supplies blood to an area of the cerebral cortex) becomes blocked by a blood clot or plaque – the region of brain concerned is immediately deprived of oxygen and nutrients, and unless blood flow can be restored quickly (within 3–4 hours) permanent brain damage will ensue. Following this, however, there is often a secondary spread of damage from the initial focus to surrounding areas. Treatment strategies have focused either on trying to restore blood flow, using clot-dissolving agents, or administering "neuroprotective "drugs to protect the surrounding brain tissue from secondary damage after the initial event. Clinical trials in stroke patients are complex and costly. In the USA a National Institutes of Health-sponsored trial of a clot-dissolving agent (tissue plasminogen activator) aimed to administer the drug to patients within 90 minutes of the stroke. The logistic difficulties of achieving this even in the USA were formidable. Such a trial could not be undertaken currently in most regions of the UK, where stroke is not treated as a medical emergency. The US trial did show a significant improvement in clinical outcome measured 3 months later, but there was also a significant increase in the occurrence of cerebral bleeding, a dangerous complication of stroke that is not easily treated. For this reason, clot-dissolving agents have not come into wide use. Other research has focused on neuroprotective strategies. One idea is that a large part of secondary damage results from the release of the neurotoxic amino acid glutamate from dead and dying brain tissue. Glutamate is normally released in small amounts as a key excitatory chemical messenger in brain, but if released in excess it causes overstimulation and death of nerve cells.

Drugs which block the excitatory effects of glutamate showed great promise as protective agents in animal models of stroke, but so far clinical trials have been disappointing. Many other refinements of this idea are under investigation, however, along with other possible neuroprotective strategies. There seems little doubt that drug regimens will be devised which can dramatically lessen the permanent brain damage which follows a stroke. The widespread introduction of such treatment regimens, however, will undoubtedly take time and be contentious, as they will be costly and will require radical changes in the medical management of stroke, with an emphasis on emergency treatment. None of the treatments can be expected to work well unless administered rapidly after the stroke. Sceptics will argue that by rescuing some people who would otherwise have died from their stroke (about one in five at the moment), the expensive new treatment may create larger numbers of permanently disabled patients who will require long-term care. On the other hand the successful treatment of stroke could lead to large numbers of patients recovering so well that they do not require long-term care. The equation will be nicely balanced, and the net outcome impossible to predict. Other protective strategies, already being assessed, rely on administering such drugs as aspirin prophylactically to protect patients known to be at risk of stroke (e.g., those who have already experienced a transient ischaemic episode ("mini-stroke") or have recovered from a stroke).

Another pharmaceutical advance that will certainly hit the headlines will be the development of safe and effective treatments for obesity. In the west obesity is an increasing public health problem, with some 20% of the British adult population classified as overweight, and the figure is closer to 30% in the USA. A large industry has grown up around dieting, with best-selling books and faddish foods. Attempts to control appetite with drugs, however, have so far proved woefully unsuccessful. The drug Redux (d-fenfluramine) proved immensely popular after its launch in the USA in 1996, but it had to be withdrawn in 1997 following alarm over reports of possibly serious heart valve abnormalities in patients taking the drug. Despite this unfortunate history, research continues unabated, and early in the twenty-first century new products will become available that will target more precisely the brain systems responsible for appetite control. In particular there will be drugs which mimic the actions of the recently discovered protein hormone leptin, which appears to act as a key link between fat tissues and appetite control centres in the brain in the control of body weight. All such interventions, however, like diets, tend to have only transient effects. When people stop taking the drugs or stop the diet, their body weight tends almost inexorably to rise again to former levels. Some scientists believe that the complex brain mechanisms involved in the control of body weight, centred in the hypothalamus, include a "set point" mechanism, i.e., if body weight goes above or below this set point it will tend automatically to readjust when conditions permit. In animals it has been known for many years that it is possible to interfere with the hypothalamic set point mechanism, either by surgical lesions or by administering selective neurotoxic drugs (e.g., gold thioglucose) which destroy some of the key nerve cells. By developing drugs which selectively target these brain centres it may be possible to provide a "one-off" treatment regimen that would permanently readjust the body weight control system downwards (or upwards in some forms of anorexia). This would create a new industry rivalling the diet business in size – and probably new lawsuits as patients complain that they are unhappy with their new body image.

Perhaps the most important advance anticipated in drug treatment of neuropsychiatric illnesses is the development of effective drugs to treat Alzheimer's disease. The twentieth century yielded some modest advances, in the form of such palliatives as Cognex (tacrine) and Aricept (donezepil), which provided some modest improvement in cognitive performance, but failed to halt the inexorable downwards progress of the disease. The real breakthroughs will come from improved understanding of the biochemical mechanisms underlying the disease process, and devising drugs which attack key parts of the disease mechanisms. The advances in identifying genetic risk factors have already strengthened the belief that a key pathological event in Alzheimer's disease is the deposition of the insoluble protein β-amyloid in brain, in the form of numerous "senile plaques". The accumulation of excess β-amyloid appears to trigger a series of events, including activation of an inflammatory response in brain, which ultimately leads to a progressive loss of nerve cells, and a consequent loss of mental function. Scientists can already see a number of targets for drug intervention to prevent excess amyloid synthesis and deposition, or even to devise drugs that might facilitate the disaggregation of existing amyloid deposits and their removal from the brain by the body's own scavenging systems. Many questions remain unanswered: How do senile plaques form? Why are they found in some areas of brain and not in others? How can patients at risk be identified before they have suffered significant brain damage and developed clinical symptoms? The research effort is now large – and the chances of success seem reasonably high. The ability to treat this appalling disease will represent a major advance – it will require great resources to achieve, but the savings in human, social and economic cost terms could be immense.

An outstanding challenge to psychopharmaceutical research remains the problem of substance abuse, including alcohol, nicotine, cocaine and other illicit drugs of various categories. Here progress to date has been modest. The best that we have to offer in the twentieth century is to substitute the drug of addiction with some safer form of the same substance. Thus, cigarette smokers use nicotine chewing gum, skin patches or inhalers to help them stop smoking; some heroin addicts find that the long-acting opiate methadone can help them over the painful withdrawal symptoms of heroin withdrawal, and maintain them in a heroin-free state. These replacement strategies, however, although better than nothing, still have a relatively poor long-term outcome. Some 90% of cigarette smokers relapse back to their habit within 12 months without treatment; those treated with nicotine still have a relapse rate of about 65%. With methadone treatment the outcome can be rather better. Scientists have not discovered any easy answers – the idea of administering blocking drugs, which prevent the pleasurable effects of the addictive drug, is theoretically attractive, and has been used successfully with the opiate antagonist naltrexone in some ex-heroin addicts. It seems possible that many drugs of addiction act through final common pathways in the brain, involving activation of both dopamine neural systems and endogenous opiates. Naltrexone, for example, has potential in the treatment of alcoholics, dissociating the pleasurable psychostimulant effects of alcohol from its sedative and antianxiety effects. But such treatments do not appeal to the great majority of addicts and are unlikely to provide any general solution.

Although substance abuse is a major social problem, it is not the case that everyone taking alcohol or even "hard" drugs is necessarily going to become addicted or have their life and career impaired. Millions of people manage to drink alcohol with minimal social cost. In other parts of the world, millions regularly use cannabis without apparent ill effects. In nineteenth century Britain the consumption of opium was widespread in all strata of society, generally without devastating consequences. It may be that in the future, genetic and behavioural screening at an early age will allow the identification of high-risk groups, those who are most likely to develop uncontrolled substance abuse. Such individuals could then be offered intensive behavioural and pharmacological treatments aimed at preventing them from becoming addicts.

Comment from Professor SH Snyder:

"In the United States 80% of all prison inmates are there because of offences that have to do one way or another with drugs. More importantly, violent crimes to a very large extent are determined by a single drug, cocaine, which stimulates paranoid anger and violence. The random killings that have made inner cities war zones can largely be attributed to cocaine. As you well know, there is virtually no treatment available for cocaine addiction despite the fact that mixed agonist-antagonists analogous to the opiate agents, would be simple to develop. For all forms of drug abuse it probably would be relatively easy to develop highly effective treatments but there is no economic incentive, and the large drug companies have done next to nothing. This is an issue that could be dealt with by governmental bodies."

New tools for monitoring brain function

The latter half of the twentieth century saw major advances in our ability to see inside the skull and examine the working of the living human brain. Neuroimaging techniques have become widely used, both as research tools and as important new aids to clinical diagnosis and monitoring. There are two main techniques, magnetic resonance imaging (MRI) and positron emission tomography (PET). In MRI the head is surrounded by a powerful magnetic field and the alignment and relaxation of water molecules in this field is measured after they are perturbed in a controlled fashion by a pulse of energy, allowing the computerised construction of a three dimensional picture of the brain. Further refinements permit the monitoring of moment to moment changes in blood flow in different brain regions, and this in turn gives a picture of which brain regions are active, because these will have the greatest blood flow.

PET uses short-lived radioactive isotopes to obtain a three dimensional picture – surrounding the head with a "camera" capable of detecting the radioactive decay events originating from inside the head. PET allows the imaging not only of cerebral blood flow (using a brief injection of radioactive water), but can also provide a chemical map of the brain by using radioactive drugs which bind selectively to those brain areas containing receptors for a particular neurotransmitter or neuropeptide. Thus, for example, one can map the distribution of dopamine receptors or opiate receptors by using suitable radiolabelled drugs.

Both MRI and PET are capable of further technical refinements – improving the spatial resolution of the measurements and shortening the time needed to complete an image. With PET it may also be possible to obtain information about the activity of particular chemical messenger systems in the brain. For example, an increased release of dopamine will displace some of the PET radiolabelled drug from binding to dopamine receptors, because both compete for these sites. In this way it should be possible to monitor the state of activity in dopamine, opiate and other chemical systems in brain, and this could provide valuable information both for the diagnosis of mental illness, or possibly for the prognosis of those at risk.

Other technologies are being assessed that could provide even more detailed information on the activity of the living brain.

Electroencephalography (EEG) has long been used to monitor the electrical activity of the brain, but it is a technique with severe limitations as it involves placing electrodes on the surface of the skull, and these can only measure the weak electrical currents that arise from the most superficial layers of the cerebral cortex. Electrical activity in the deeper structures of the brain cannot be measured in this way. This problem can be overcome, however, by the technique of magnetoencephalography (MEG), which measures not the electrical currents generated by the electrical activity of nerve cells, but the minute changes in magnetic field which arise from such activity. The magnetic field changes can be registered by an array of very sensitive sensors placed around the head, and by using computerised tomography it is possible to build up a three-dimensional picture of the electrical activity of all parts of the brain – not just its surface. The technical problems here remain formidable, and relate in large part to how to handle the mass of data generated by this technique. Brain cells may fire electrical impulses several hundred times per second, and in principle MEG could provide data on brain activity with a millisecond timeframe, – rather than the time resolution of existing techniques in tens of seconds or minutes. Advances in computerised data handling will no doubt help to overcome such problems.

One could envisage a diagnostic screening of brain function in the future, using a combination of imaging techniques to assess electrical activity and chemical status that might help pinpoint malfunctions in particular brain systems before these become manifest in clinical symptoms of disease. Such screening is already possible, although not widely used. By using repeated PET imaging and a radiolabelled drug fluoro-DOPA that enters the brain and is converted to fluoro-dopamine in dopamine-rich brain areas, the progression of Parkinson's disease can be monitored as these brain regions gradually degenerate. One could imagine using such a screen every few years after the age of 55 to detect the earliest stages of the disease, and then intervening immediately with implant surgery to boost the population of dopamine neurons before any symptoms of the illness become apparent. This "Brave New World" scenario is already virtually within our grasp. Initially though this will only be medicine for the rich, as the costs of large-scale screening of this type will be beyond present-day health system resources. But the rich man's medicine may eventually become commonplace as screening methods improve and costs are reduced.

Further reading

Clauw DJ, Chrousos GP. Chronic pain and fatigue syndromes: overlapping clinical and neuroendocrine features and potential pathogenic mechanisms. *Neuroimmunomodulation* 1997; **4**: 134–53.

Cooper JR, Bloom FE, Roth RH. *The Biochemical Basis of Neuropharmacology*, 7th edn. Oxford University Press, New York, 1996.

Dunnett SB, Kendall AL, Watts C, Torres EM. Neuronal cell transplantation for Parkinson's and Huntington's diseases. *Brit Med Bull* 1997; **53**: 757–76.

Flier JS. Leptin expression and action: new experimental paradigms. *Proc Natl Acad Sci USA* 1997; **94**: 4240–5.

Healy D. The antidepressant era. Harvard University Press, Cambridge, MA, 1997.

Institute of Medicine. *Pathways of addiction. Opportunities in drug abuse research*. National Academy Press, Washington DC, 1996.

Jennings C. How trinucleotide repeats may function. *Nature* 1995; **378**: 127.

Martinez-Serrano A, Björklund A. Immortalized neural progenitor cells for CNS gene transfer and repair. *Trends Neurosci* 1997; **20**: 530–7.

Nainggolan L. Xenotransplantation – saving our bacon? *Scrip Magazine* 1996; **December**: 38–42.

Nainggolan L. Slow progress in the treatment of stroke. *Scrip Magazine* 1998; **March**: 29–32.

Olson L. Regeneration in the adult nervous system: experimental repair strategies. *Nature Med* 1997; **3**: 1329–35.

Selkoe DJ. Alzheimer's disease: genotypes, phenotypes and treatments. *Science*, 1997; **275**: 630–1.

The following colleagues were invited to act as commentators on early drafts:

Alexandra Wyke
Managing Editor, Economist Intelligence Unit, London, UK

Professor SH Snyder
Department of Neuroscience, Johns Hopkins University School of Medicine, Baltimore MD, USA

Professor Richard SJ Frackowiak
Wellcome Department of Cognitive Neurology, Institute of Neurology, University of London, London, UK

Professor Anders Björklund
Wallenberg Neurocentrum, Institut Fysiologi, Neurovetenskap, Solvegaten, Sweden

Dr George Kobb
Department of Neuropharmacology, Scripps Research Institute, La Jolla, USA

6 The heart and circulation

Philip Poole-Wilson

> Wood chopping is so popular because you can see the results of your activity immediately
>
> Albert Einstein

Introduction

Predicting the direction of future change is the privilege of the more elderly, while the young often unknowingly are responsible for change. And predictions can so easily be wrong. As George Eliot put it: "Of all errors prophecy is the most pernicious". Prophecy can be used to justify almost any intended action. That has not inhibited many persons and often those in positions of considerable influence wallowing in the authoritarian joys of fantasy with regard to the future direction of science and research. In general the medical profession has been largely devoid of this transgression. But economists and politicians, for example, often impose their perception of the future with almost no evidence for the consequences other than the belief that what is proposed is better or, at least, different from the current situation. Government has adopted a different approach with regard to science. Foresight analysis, a methodology intended to minimise the arbitrary nature of decision making, has become a popular management tool but has many limitations. It is in reality little more than the consensual expression of expert opinions on the direction of the future so that if that vision is wrong, those responsible will be in good company and no doubt have many excuses at the ready and well prepared. Inevitably, like foresight analysis, this chapter will consist of guesses, speculation, and erroneous future scenarios.

The scientific and social environment

Recent events in medicine must lead to concern that the control of key areas of influence will limit future developments. For example a reduction in the number of truly independent medical schools and the formation of rigid groupings within medical schools will inevitably diminish the opportunity for original research to appear and flourish. The enthusiasm for large inter-disciplinary units in the belief that such a system will encourage scientific advance is not based on a substantial body of evidence. Indeed many of the successful units in the last HEFCE assessment of research in the UK were focused units. Many of the most famous medical institutions in this country owe their reputation to the fact that those institutions have been allowed to flourish and bring together expertise on a focused topic rather than suffering from the inevitable dilution of effort in a large organisation covering all topics in a more general manner. The problem does not only exist in universities and medical schools. Most major funding bodies are increasingly concentrating their resources on fewer but larger research units. Heads of scientific laboratories or institutes have more authority than previously to determine or even impose the direction of research. Such very large groupings have not always been notable for their success. True innovation may be snuffed out by these monoliths.

Perhaps our greatest danger lies in the poor level of scientific education, which is evident in persons who have authority over the control and governance of science. There is an urgent need to improve the knowledge of science in the population at large, but in particular among politicians, economists, managers, and administrators. This will take a generation, or possibly longer, because the problem lies in the schools and the limited education in science which is received by so many who go on to be in positions of authority in this country.

Cardiovascular medicine is a changing subject and is not immune to the pressures that society is now imposing on scientists. Whatever doubts may exist concerning the validity of current fashion in the organisation of research, the public demand for accountability of expenditure will make it essential for every scientist and research institute to have a clear plan of their purpose. That strategy will be needed not to promote the best science but rather to satisfy the perceived needs of managers, politicians, and the public. The imposition of the need to explain the what and why of an activity is not conducive to the promotion of originality and innovation. The direction of research should not be led by dogma but by new science. There can be only one genuine reason for beholding the crystal ball and considering the future and that is because it is fun and satisfying; necessity and correctness are secondary.

A further factor in determining the future of science is the problem of financial reward. Traditionally in this country the scientist has been stigmatised as a highly intelligent person, pursuing knowledge for its own sake, not desirous of the luxuries of life, and with an unrealistic appreciation of the financial world. The scientist is not perceived as streetwise. That is about to change. The opportunity to patent inventions and discoveries and the realisation that the achievements of the scientist are not as appreciated as those of the manager, administrator or politician, will lead to scientists seeking to sell their skills at a rate compatible with those of other entrepreneurs or professionals in society.

History and recent achievements

The last 40 years has seen nothing less than a total transformation of the treatment of most cardiovascular diseases. The introduction of the thiazide diuretics in 1958 was perhaps the greatest milestone in cardiovascular medicine of this century. A little later the powerful loop diuretics became available. This group of drugs, known as diuretics, has allowed physicians to control and manipulate the total sodium and water content of the body. These drugs transformed the treatment of heart failure but were also useful in the management of renal disease, liver disease and high blood pressure where fluid retention remains part of the clinical problem. In the 1960s Sir James Black was responsible for the introduction of beta-blockers into clinical practice. These drugs inhibit the effects of activation of the sympathetic system in the body. Beta-blockers were soon shown, as predicted, to be of clinical benefit in patients with angina pectoris and hypertension. More recently there has been some enthusiasm for using these drugs in the treatment of heart failure, because activation of the sympathetic system is the earliest body response to weakness of the heart and sympathetic activation may be harmful by increasing the rate at which the contractile cells (myocytes) in the heart die.

More recently four groups of drugs have assumed immense importance. Aspirin has been shown to be of benefit in patients with acute myocardial infarction and has a role in the prevention of the progression of coronary heart disease. Thrombolytic drugs, "clot busters", were introduced for the treatment of acute myocardial infarction which was shown to be due to instability of an atheromatous plaque in the coronary artery associated with the development of thrombosis (clot formation). These drugs were shown to reduce the in-hospital and short-term mortality from myocardial infarction. The benefit has now been shown to persist over time. The angiotensin converting enzyme (ACE) inhibitors were introduced to inhibit the activation of the renin–angiotensin system. The renin–angiotensin system, like the sympathetic system, is a hormonal mechanism built into the body and designed to be of advantage to the human when under conditions of stress such as exercise, fluid deprivation, and haemorrhage. The system is activated inappropriately when patients have some forms of heart disease. ACE inhibitors have been shown to reduce mortality and morbidity in patients with almost any form of heart failure. Finally the group of drugs known as statins has recently been introduced to lower cholesterol. Cholesterol is a major risk factor for coronary heart disease. This group of drugs has been shown to reduce mortality, morbidity, hospitalisation and medical procedures in patients with coronary heart disease. Thus in cardiovascular medicine the impact of new drugs cannot be underestimated. Nor should the fact that much of this research was undertaken in the pharmaceutical industry be overlooked. Most of these discoveries would not have been brought to fruition without successful cooperation between scientists, universities, clinicians, and industry.

At the same time there have been great advances based on technology rather than therapeutics. In relation to heart disease perhaps the most important has been the development of small reliable and sophisticated pacemakers. These are used not only to treat patients in whom the heart has lost its natural ability to beat but also to control abnormal rhythms of the heart. More recently devices known as intracardiac cardioverter defibrillators (ICDs) have become available. These devices give the heart a small electric shock from electrodes connected by wires to an an implanted box. The device is used in patients whose hearts have a tendency to develop abnormal rhythms that may lead to sudden death. The design and manufacture of artificial heart valves has developed. Not only are there improved mechanical artificial valves but also biological valves where the material is obtained either from pigs or from humans.

It has long been the ambition of man to produce an artificial heart. The programme undertaken in the USA was not successful, or at least not yet after several decades, but there are now available artificial devices which have been shown to maintain humans alive for periods of up to 1 year prior to transplantation. New artificial pumps to assist the function of the heart are being developed.

By far the most widely used treatment based on technology has been the design of small wires, catheters, balloons, and stents. These are all devices by which tubes can be placed into the arterial system of humans through a small puncture usually of the femoral artery. The tubes can be manipulated and advanced to almost anywhere in the circulation but particularly into the coronary arteries (the arteries arising from the aorta and supplying the blood to heart muscle). Miniaturisation has led to a vast array of gadgets, which can be placed on the ends of these catheters, such as cutting devices, laser systems, devices for delivery of radiation, echocardiographic systems for visualisation of the artery wall or direct visualisation of the inner surface of the artery. Initially balloons on the ends of these catheters were available, which could be blown up externally and used to open up obstructions in coronary arteries by simply pressurising the narrowing and tearing the tissue apart (percutaneous transluminal coronary angioplasty, PTCA). Later developments resulted in stents made of various materials in a panoply of designs, which could then hold the artery, widely open. More recently some of these devices have been designed to deliver radiation or drugs which are impregnated on the surface of the stents.

The availability of new drugs, the advances in engineering technology and the development of human transplantation have been the spur to the progress, which has been made in cardiovascular medicine over the last 40 years. The future in cardiovascular medicine is a race between the potential of technology and the opportunities presented by the new biology.

Epidemiological inevitability

For the next 20 years, at least, cardiovascular disease is going to be the major cause of death and medical disability in the world. Such a statement is not a hopeful prediction from those, like myself with a vested interest, but a racing certainty. The major cardiovascular disease is called ischaemic heart disease (or perhaps more accurately coronary heart disease). This is caused by the development of atheromatous plaques in the arterial wall of the coronary arteries. These plaques can break down spontaneously, initiate thrombosis, obstruct the artery and cause a myocardial infarction (heart attack). Alternatively the plaques increase in size so limiting the passage of blood to the muscle of the heart causing angina. The spectrum of the clinical consequences of atheromatous plaques are angina, unstable angina, heart attacks, sudden death, or heart failure. The development of atheroma is slow and takes place over many years. Many persons who now regard themselves as healthy will have extensive atheroma in the coronary arteries. WHO in conjunction with the World Bank and Harvard University has recently published an authoritative study of diseases in the entire world divided into groupings such as developed and developing nations. Their prediction is that by the year 2020 the five major causes of death will be ischaemic heart disease, cerebrovascular disease, chronic obstructive pulmonary disorders, lower tract respiratory infections and diseases of the trachea, bronchus and lungs (Figure 6.1). The major causes of morbidity or disability

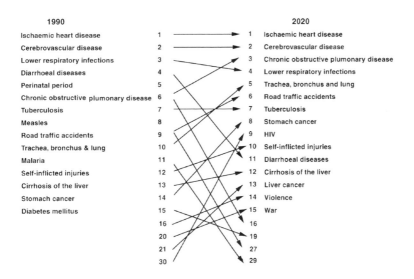

Figure 6.1 Rank order for the overall cause of death in the world 1990–2020. By the year 2020 it is predicted that heart disease, vascular disease and lung disease will be the major health problems in the world. The pattern is rather similar for developed and developing countries. (Reproduced from Murray and Lopez.[1])

measured in disability adjusted life years (DALYS) will be ischaemic heart disease, unipolar depression, road traffic accidents, cerebrovascular disease, and chronic obstructive lung disorders (Figure 6.2). The pattern of disease will be rather similar in both developed and developing countries. This is a major change and implies that the importance of infectious disorders such as malaria and diarrhoeal diseases will diminish. Chronic disorders such as ischaemic heart disease will become more prominent worldwide.

At first sight such evidence may appear rather depressing, but the reasons for these expectations are important to understand. Two major changes, one in medical practice and one in demography, are critical. The first is that in the last 40 years the management and treatment of cardiovascular disorders has improved greatly. In addition there have been major advances in prevention. Thus coronary heart disease in middle age is falling in most western countries and there has been a very substantial increase in overall life expectancy (Figure 6.3). Partly this has been the consequence of therapeutic intervention and partly because of changes in social circumstances such as the alleviation of chronic illness, social deprivation, life dissatisfaction, and poor nourishment. Nevertheless, the fact that in most countries there has been

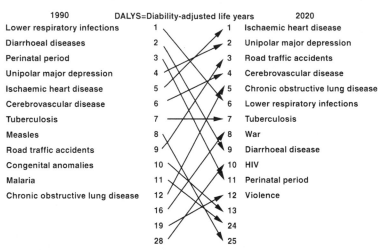

1990		DALYS=Diability-adjusted life years		2020
Lower respiratory infections	1		1	Ischaemic heart disease
Diarrhoeal diseases	2		2	Unipolar major depression
Perinatal period	3		3	Road traffic accidents
Unipolar major depression	4		4	Cerebrovascular disease
Ischaemic heart disease	5		5	Chronic obstructive lung disease
Cerebrovascular disease	6		6	Lower respiratory infections
Tuberculosis	7		7	Tuberculosis
Measles	8		8	War
Road traffic accidents	9		9	Diarrhoeal disease
Congenital anomalies	10		10	HIV
Malaria	11		11	Perinatal period
Chronic obstructive lung disease	12		12	Violence
	16		13	
	19		24	
	28		25	

Figure 6.2 The major causes of the burden of disease measured in terms of disability-adjusted life years will in 2020 be ischaemic heart disease, depression, and road traffic accidents. Vascular and lung diseases will also be important. The significance of infective disorders will diminish. (Reproduced from Murray and Lopez.[1])

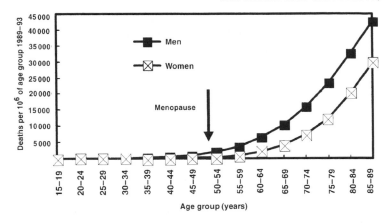

Figure 6.3   Deaths from ischaemic heart disease by age group in the UK for the years 1989–93. For women the increase with age lags about 10 years behind men. (Drawn from data taken from Tunstall-Pedoc.[2])

a reduction in the mortality in the critical age range of 45–65 years has meant that more persons live to a greater age where they may be afflicted by the same disease entity or other diseases. The second consideration is related to the first and is that the demographic distribution of persons within western countries is and will change dramatically (Figure 6.4). Most western countries and developing countries have a predominance of young persons in their popula-

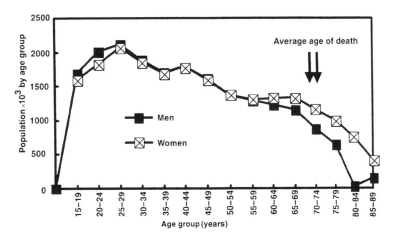

Figure 6.4   The distribution of the population by age in the UK in the years 1989–93. (Drawn from data taken from Tunstall-Pedoc.[2])

tion. With the improvement of health care this pattern will change so that by the year 2020 there will be a greater proportion of elderly persons in the population. This is inevitable and is a change which is entirely predictable. The demographic change has some rather startling consequences. Although the rate of death in younger age groups from cardiovascular diseases such as heart attacks and stroke will diminish, the total number of persons with heart attacks, stroke or heart failure in the overall population may increase. That is because the reduction of the occurrence of these entities in the young is offset by an increase in the occurrence in the elderly. Ischaemic heart disease, strokes and heart failure are diseases of the elderly. Even if in the elderly the rate of these events is reduced the total number of persons experiencing such an event will increase because the total number of persons in that age group will increase. A good example is the prevalence of heart failure in Australia (Figure 6.5). Thus cardiovascular medicine will continue to be a major entity in the delivery of health care but the patients who are being treated will be in the more elderly group.

Epidemiology and risk factors for cardiovascular disease

Epidemiology includes the study of those factors which contribute to the development of a chronic disease such as heart attacks or strokes. The last 20 years has witnessed many large studies in different countries. It is now possible to make a comparison of

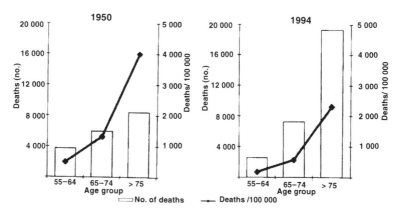

Figure 6.5 Number of deaths and mortality rate from coronary heart disease in Australia in 1950 and 1994. (Reproduced from Kelly.[3])

known risk factors between different countries, within countries, and within identifiable subgroups in countries. The argument has then been put that if such factors can be identified their prevention would inevitably result in major benefit to the community. The major risk factors for coronary heart disease have been shown to be smoking, lipid abnormalities (abnormalities of blood fat and raised cholesterol), hypertension (high blood pressure), diabetes, obesity, and lack of exercise. There are in addition innumerable other factors, which are related in some small way to the occurrence of cardiovascular events. These include a whole spectrum of factors, some coming close to being "old wives' tales". Thus there is hard and soft water, personality, stress, hormones, wine drinking, and place of abode. Most of these so-called risk factors are very minor determinants of the likelihood of a person developing coronary heart disease. Recently the emphasis has shifted to new risk factors such as birth weight and circumstances surrounding childhood, metabolic factors such as the blood level of homocysteine or fibrinogen, poverty and social deprivation, and finally what has been called decision latitude. Many experts have for long thought that personality and a sense of achievement are related to the occurrence of coronary heart disease. Decision latitude is a phrase used to identify the unresolved conflict represented by undesired circumstances and the inability to influence or change those circumstances. For example, persons who are in a repetitive and dull job and who are unable to alter their circumstances because of the need for financial gain, have a lack of decision latitude compared to those who have what is perceived as a more agreeable job and are able to alter the nature of their work pattern to optimise the satisfaction obtained from work.

In the next two decades there will be major changes in the approach to the prediction of coronary heart disease. The major error in the past has been the emphasis that has been placed on individual risk factors. None of these risk factors are sufficiently powerful to have great impact when applied singly to populations or communities. Groups have formed, and even medical societies, which specialise in the reversal of a single risk factor. For example there are pressure groups and societies with regard to smoking, abnormal levels of fat and cholesterol, and above all the treatment of hypertension. Hypertension is a word used to describe the blood pressure, which is measured in millimetres of mercury. A high blood pressure is associated with an increased incidence of stroke and coronary heart disease. It is odd to have scientific or medical societies, which are related to a measurement and not a disease outcome. Undoubtedly the word hypertension implies mistakenly the existence of a disease entity rather than of a measurement, which is made with a blood cuff being placed around the arm. Hypertension is perceived as a disease and not as a risk factor for several disease outcomes.

The concept of global risk is being developed. Information obtained from communities within towns, within countries and within continents will allow more accurate predictions to be made by the entry of say 20–50 variables into a computer program. This will result in more accurate identification of who is at risk, who is not and what interventions might maximise the ability to change that risk. It will be possible to keep this information on individual persons or patients on small individualised data cards.

Undoubtedly new risk factors will emerge as the nature of the origins and pathology of coronary events are better understood. In addition there are considerable hopes for genetics. At present the public is concerned about genetics because of a fear that it may reveal the inner secrets of their body or even their mind. On the other hand the role of genetics has long been known and used in medicine. Simple questions such as the occurrence of a disease entity in relatives or the age of death of one's parents have at their root a genetic origin. Many genetic abnormalities are being identified which do relate to the tendency of an individual person to develop coronary heart disease. At present the importance of these factors is greatly exaggerated. The genetic makeup of the human body is so complex (over 100 000 genes) that current research can only be regarded as tinkering at the edges. In 20 years' time a simple sample of blood, a skin scraping or a sample of saliva will allow the identification in moments of many hundred gene variations which will be added to the common known risk factors for coronary heart disease and added to an individual's data card. This will be perceived as an entirely normal procedure of benefit to mankind and unwarranted fears will be put aside as the benefits become only too evident. Some genes may bring an advantage to a population. For example a gene which limits the need for salt in areas where salt is difficult to come by, such as the desert, could be beneficial. But the price to pay is that when salt becomes freely available following so-called development that same gene leads to disorders such as hypertension. This possibility is known as the "thrifty gene" hypothesis and variations of the argument could account for differences, which seem to exist between populations in the prevalence of certain risk factors and the response to particular risk factors for coronary heart disease.

Objectives of a health policy or a medical treatment

Health policies and the introduction of new medical or surgical treatments should be driven by their impact on precisely defined objectives. The purpose of medicine is to prevent the occurrence of disease, prolong life and improve the quality of life by minimising unwanted symptoms. There are no other objectives. Where treatments are to be introduced which impact on large groups of patients then it will be necessary to demonstrate benefit in terms of these three criteria. In the past that has not always been so. For example in the treatment of hypertension and the lowering of cholesterol, drugs have been licensed because they lower blood pressure and cholesterol and it has been presumed that that reduction will be a surrogate for benefit in terms of major objectives. That argument can no longer be sustained in general. In future it will be a requirement that measures of outcome are shown to be improved by an intervention, not just the expected biological impact. Numerous examples exist where surrogate end-points have not been demonstrated to be advantageous. Several drugs are known to improve central haemodynamics and exercise capacity in patients with heart failure and yet these very same drugs lead to an increase in mortality. Conversely some drugs which improve mortality may impact unfavourably on surrogate end-points. There will be an increasing need for all treatments, especially those directed towards many persons in the community, to be tested fully before their general introduction. In small groups of patients with specific diseases such an approach is impractical and surrogate end-points will continue to be the standard by which outcome is assessed.

Perception of life

The objectives of health policy are closely related to the perception by the public of the most acceptable pattern of life. Health policy is usually a political decision to which doctors make a small contribution. In recent years there has been an increasing expectation that medicine can reverse or resolve almost any

131

affliction to which man is susceptible. Achievements are emphasised more than limitations. Over the next 20–50 years that concept will be reversed and there will be a sharper distinction between the expectation of the public and the reality of what can be delivered. At present many sections of the public expect only perfection and success from the medical profession and any failure is a matter for litigation. The individual expects but carries too little responsibility for their own actions or their participation in decisions. The rights of individual persons will increase in the next decades, but so will the responsibility of individuals and the acceptance of risk associated with medical decisions agreed between patient and doctor.

This problem is exemplified by the current possibilities in the treatment of heart failure. At present there are a series of drugs such as diuretics, ACE inhibitors and possibly beta-blockers which have been shown to prolong life in patients with this unpleasant disease. However, much of the last few years of life of patients with heart failure is miserable because of severe disabling and limiting symptoms. There are several drugs which have been shown to improve these symptoms but to reduce the duration of life. For that reason these drugs have been withdrawn from the market and are not available to the public. The decision to disallow the use of these drugs has been made by drug authorities set up in individual countries and not by the patient, the public, governments, or even doctors. Most persons in an ideal world would prefer to live for a long period of time with a high quality of life. That is what might be called the square wave of life. What is to be avoided is early or premature death or prolonged debilitating disease over many years leading to death. There is thus a decision to be made with regard to the degree to which medical intervention might improve symptoms at the cost of diminishing duration of life. Those are decisions which in the future should be made by patients and doctors within the limitations set by government.

To many lay people it will be surprising that the medical profession is often unable to describe precisely the mode of death of human beings. It is a truism that all persons eventually die because the heart stops beating. Society has acknowledged that if the brain ceases to function the body may be described as dead regardless of the fact that the heart and lungs may be functioning in a limited state. Those organs can then be used for transplantation. Most people have an abhorrence of a long drawn out and painful death. I return to the concept of the square wave of life

132

where death is sudden at a great age. In future years there will be much emphasis on research into the mode of death and the circumstances surrounding death. Even simple information is often not available such as the place of death, the time of death, the last occasion when the person was seen well, the validity of information on death certificates, and the validity of information even after a post-mortem examination. The accuracy of death certificates across the world is poor. Often persons are labelled as having for example coronary heart disease because that is a sociably acceptable cause of death. If such data is then placed in national statistics gross errors can arise. Even post-mortem examinations do not always reveal the cause of death. That is particularly so if death is due to a physiological event such as spasm of a coronary artery or an artery supplying the brain leading to a restriction of function for a short period of time and then to death. The patterns of death in patients with cancer, AIDS, and terminal heart failure are somewhat similar. The cachexia which is associated with these disorders is currently being investigated and drugs will surely become available to alter and prevent the onset or at least the progression of cachexia.

Prevention

The concept of the prevention of disease has been promoted particularly by the epidemiologists for some time and to some extent has become a mantra. No one could possibly argue that prevention is not the most desirable objective and that has been demonstrated in particular for infectious diseases. The issue becomes rather more confused when the well-known phrase "prevention is better than cure" is changed to "prevention rather than cure" as in *The Times* newspaper in 1979. Many persons would be concerned if when they presented themselves at hospital with chest pain, possibly indicating a heart attack, they were to be informed all resources had been spent on prevention and that the acute episode could not be managed. Nevertheless it is an important concept that ever-increasing expenditure on the obvious end-points of coronary heart disease may limit expenditure which could prevent at least some of those episodes occurring. Far too much of current medical resources are spent on health care in the last year of life. Those who favour prevention may promote the cynical view that cardiologists and specialists merely deal with the failures of others to prevent disease.

The demonstration that prevention is effective in coronary heart disease has not been that simple to establish. Certainly age-related deaths from coronary heart disease are falling in the UK and in many other countries (Figure 6.6). That could be due to preventive measures or to medical treatment or to some undeclared change in a determinant of the aetiology of atheromatous obstruction in the coronary arteries. The latter is the underlying pathophysiology which leads to heart attacks. On the other hand some major studies of prevention have shown that the implementation of preventive measures in Europe is poor and that even when considerable money and effort is put into prevention it is difficult to demonstrate a benefit in terms of outcome. The failure to demonstrate a benefit may be because of the lack of power of studies. Huge numbers of healthy persons need to be studied in order to demonstrate a reduction in a disease entity which, although the major cause of death in middle age, will only affect a small proportion of the total number in that age group.

For the future preventive measures will need to be more focused. This will be achieved by the use of more extensive information to establish a risk profile in an individual patient and more information with regard to the significance and interactions between combinations of risk factors. That will in turn depend upon advances in information technology.

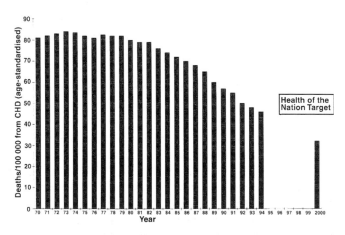

Figure 6.6   Age-standardised death rates from coronary heart disease in England: age group 16–64 years. (Reproduced from Department of Health.[4])

Fetal and paediatric biology and cardiovascular medicine

In recent years a hypothesis has been put forward which has come to be known as the Barker hypothesis that events during pregnancy and in the neonatal period may influence the tendency of persons to develop coronary heart disease in later life. The mechanisms may be many and include not just a biological mechanisms but issues such as social deprivation, housing, and the cost of food. Were that to be so then improvements in social circumstances should lead to a reduction in coronary heart disease. That is indeed one explanation of the reductions in persons of middle age which have been observed. The consequence is that health policies might be more directed towards social deprivation and poverty rather than to a specific medical intervention.

The last 20 years have seen spectacular advances in paediatric cardiology and the ability to treat although not cure many complex disorders of the heart. Many abnormalities can now be detected during pregnancy and there is the possibility that as genetic abnormalities associated with many of these disorders are established it will be possible to make the diagnosis at an even earlier stage. Whatever the moral approach to termination may be, that is an option, particularly in healthy young couples, for the prevention of the birth of children with such abnormalities. A better approach in families at risk is perhaps to identify at an early stage ova which do not contain the abnormal gene pattern and to allow parents to give birth to a child without the propensity to induce these known abnormalities. Undoubtedly this approach is going to develop substantially in the next 40 years so that the role of paediatric cardiology in treating heart disorders will diminish.

Scientific base

Activities in cardiovascular medicine in the next five decades will be greatly influenced by advances in biology. In particular the further understanding of the processes involved in atheroma should lead to a variety of new treatments. At present there is enthusiasm for reducing cholesterol and there are a number of hypotheses concerning the activation of biological systems for the breakdown of the structure of the atheromatous plaque and at the same time a reduction in those processes which are expected to stabilise a plaque. The majority of the current biology is descriptive. Relating research findings to clinical outcome in terms of

135

important events such as heart attacks or the progression of angina has not been achieved. Closely linked to future work in atheroma is the current enthusiasm for the function of the endothelium. A controversial projection is that most of the current work on atheroma will turn out to be a description of the events on the way to disorganisation and death of accumulated smooth muscle cells and that new work will provide more evidence on the fundamental links between risk factors and those biological factors initiating the damage to the atheromatous wall. The function of the endothelium will be shown to control and balance the flow of blood through tissues and not to be a major determinant of flow itself or of the function of the particular organ. In the next two decades advances will be limited to those processes which initiate atheroma, lead to instability of the plaque and impact on clotting and thrombosis and on known risk factors rather than on the new biology.

To bring about major changes in the circulation requires the generation of new vessels. Recently there have been reports claiming to show that the insertion of certain peptides into the muscle of the heart promoted the development of new blood vessels to the heart. This direction of research is likely to prove fruitful and indeed in years to come the treatment of angina pectoris may be not by cardiac surgery but by the insertion of substances in a controlled manner through needles or laser channels, utilising minimally invasive surgery and not requiring the chest to be opened.

The second key area for development is cardiac transplantation and the promotion of cell growth or hyperplasia. Considerable interest surrounds the future of xenotransplantation. Some of the problems of acute rejection have been overcome but there is little evidence that delayed and chronic rejection will not remain a major problem. In addition there is the possibility that the pig heart could be the vector for transmission of undesirable viruses into the human genome. Although undoubtedly xenotransplantation will be undertaken, I am doubtful whether it will become a major method for the treatment of terminal heart failure; that may be more influenced by the development of new mechanical devices.

An alternative to xenotransplantation is cell transplantation. Either agents or genes could be developed which would bring about division or at least separation of the human myocardial cell or cells could be grown in culture and seeded or inserted into the human myocardium. The current dogma is that the number of cells in the human heart is fixed soon after birth. There has always been a literature which has countered that claim. Approximately 20% of cells in the human myocardium contain two nuclei (multiple nuclei) and some cells have double the DNA in one nucleus (polyploidy). There is therefore the possibility that the number of cells in the human heart could increase to a limited extent by the separation of the two nuclei in any single cell to form two cells. A means will be found to control the growth of the cell both to increase the growth and to decrease the growth. The seeding of cultured cells into the myocardium will certainly develop and be a major treatment within 40 years. Cells will be cultured from neonatal human and animal tissue. The precursor cells of other cell types such as smooth muscle cells or fibroblasts will be used to create myocardial cells for transfer into the heart. Heart transplantation will become not organ transplantation but cell transplantation.

Much hope has been generated with regard to the process of gene transfer. More recently there has been a diminution in the enthusiasm for this process. My enthusiasm remains totally undiminished. The major problems which exist such as the means of transferring the gene to the cell, the dose of gene to be delivered, the duration of action of the gene can be resolved and represent not scientific blocks to progress but technical problems which will not be beyond the wit of man to overcome. The heart represents a particularly attractive organ in which to initiate experiments on gene transfer. At present there are innumerable techniques which can deliver genes into the coronary arteries. It is a simple matter to insert drugs into the myocardium, either at the time of surgery or using minimally invasive techniques such as laser-created channels in the myocardium or direct injection with a needle. The pericardium provides a useful space surrounding the heart into which genes or gene vehicles could be inserted and removed over a known time period. There is a lack of work at the moment on the effectiveness of delivery if drugs or any gene product were to be placed in the pericardial space. A further advantage of studying patients with heart disease is that some patients particularly those with severe coronary heart disease or severe heart failure, are known to have a poor prognosis. Issues such as the risk of developing cancer are almost totally irrelevant in such circumstances.

The third major innovative advance will be in the area of genetics. There are many polymorphisms, which are now thought to predict some aspects of coronary heart disease. Genetic abnormalities have been identified as a cause for several cardiac conditions including hypertrophic cardiomyopathy, arrhythmias, cardiac malformations and even some rare forms of idiopathic dilated cardiomyopathy. Not only will there be the identification of many more genetic abnormalities associated with cardiovascular disease but characterising the genetic profile of patients will allow treatment to be directed in a more effective manner. The use of genetic information to determine therapy of patients will develop rapidly in the next decade.

Technological base

The advances in biology and the understanding of pathophysiology have rather overshadowed the advances that technology has provided to cardiology. Examples at present are the use of stents to open up coronary arteries after angioplasty, the availability of intracardiac cardioverter defibrillators, the development of small left ventricular assist devices using centrifugal pumps, and the possibility of using mechanical structures for tissue engineering. All these techniques are going to advance in a spectacular fashion. Within the next few years perfusion pumps will become available which can be inserted into the apex of the left ventricle and directly into the aorta. These will be eventually inserted through a small incision and it will be possible to remove them if and when the myocardium recovers in response to other treatments. The devices will be powered by new battery sources and coils will be available so that electrical power can be passed through the skin to the internal pump. The function of the pump will be under computer control and totally adjustable according to the biological needs of the body estimated from a variety of biological sensors. Even the characteristics of the pump, such as the angle of the leading edge on a centrifugal pump, will be under computer control.

Stents are at present made of simple materials to fairly standard designs. Stents could be made in a way so that the shape of the stent reacts to the movement of the heart and to the movement of the vessel. Energy can be stored in that way. It is also probable that stents will open and close according to the requirement for blood flow and even deliver drugs according to need.

Devices for the treatment of ventricular tachycardia and ventricular fibrillation will be transformed by the development of new electrode systems which are able to detect the abnormal pathways across the heart and to insert electrical impulses at particular sites in order to block the electrical pathways which initiate ventricular tachycardia. This will obviate the need for ICDs, which will continue to be developed for the next ten years. Electrical instability of the heart will be a problem largely solved unless it is associated with the progression of gross disease.

Tissue engineering will advance consequent upon a combination of biological and technological expertise. Artificial materials will be developed upon which biological cells can be cultured and grown. This will provide new valves and new blood vessels, particularly for the few remaining patients who will still need to undergo coronary artery bypass grafting. The use of vein grafts will become totally redundant, avoiding the unpleasant consequences of removing the veins from the legs.

Communications and information technology

A major advance in cardiovascular medicine will develop from the growth in communications in information technology. Telemedicine will result in a major revolution and this will be led by cardiovascular medicine. Primary, secondary and tertiary centres will be closely linked. It will be possible to transmit the physiognomy of the patient with all investigations instantly between doctors and specialists. Even consultations will occur at considerable distance. The medical records of patients including X-rays, electrocardiograms and echocardiograms will be placed on smart cards which can be inserted in specialised devices and transmitted to relevant doctors. These same techniques will impact in a major way on education and teaching and on the dissemination of knowledge to the public. The current concern with privacy will be resolved by technology but also because of a change in the public attitude as the advantages of computerisation of records become evident.

One casualty of this system will be the conventional medical journal. It will not be sustainable for editors and publishing companies who profit greatly from current medical journals to maintain the argument that they should be the arbitrators of good science through the refereeing system. Information will be transmitted through known channels over the internet and publications will have comments and criticisms attached using that system. There will be guards against uninformed criticism. The role of editors and referees will move in the direction of becoming keepers of the system rather than towards pontification and decision making over what constitutes important science. After all if a publication is so dull or of such poor quality that no one wants to access the information on the internet, it could be cast into the lower dungeons in the encyclopedia of knowledge while papers of interest could be allowed to bask longer in the upper regions of current knowledge.

Trials

The randomised control trial has become the gold standard for the evaluation of any form of treatment in medicine, be it either a trial of a new medicine, or a new surgical technique. The proper design of trials has become almost a speciality in its own right. A crucial point that has been emphasised again and again is that trials must have the appropriate power to determine a change in an outcome measure which is defined in size and has clinical relevance. A trial also should have power so that the demonstration of no difference between two treatments does indicate that in reality there is no clinically relevant benefit from the putative new treatment. Because trials have often been too small, meta-analysis was developed as a mathematical technique for assessing the outcome from several trials. The technique has considerable advantages but also disadvantages in that trials may be different in design, of different duration, and include patients with different initial characteristics. Putting such information together may lead to errors. Undoubtedly the randomised clinical trial will remain the gold standard for some time but the limitations of meta-analysis will become better understood.

A key problem with the randomised controlled trial is that the trial is inevitably undertaken on particular groups of patients who can be identified by doctors and who agree to participate in that trial. The outcome gives no indication of effect in those who refuse to participate in a trial or on patients outside the inclusion criteria of a trial. There are some key examples of this problem in medical practice at the present time. If we were to keep rigidly to the mantra of evidence-based medicine many people would not receive particular types of treatment. What a patient requests is not evidence-based medicine but patient-based evidence; that is the patient wishes to know whether that particular form of treatment will be of benefit to them as an individual. The answer to that question is rarely possible in cardiovascular medicine. What clinicians commonly do is apply the results of clinical trials to groups of patients not included in the original trial on the basis of other evidence supporting the notion that the indications for the treatment can be broadened from the limited inclusion criteria of the initial study.

That approach will no longer be acceptable in the future. Another solution is to obtain large databases after clinical trials have demonstrated initial efficacy. Newer mathematical approaches will be developed which will utilise large databases so as to determine whether benefit accrues in all subsets of patients. The formation of these databases will be aided by the development of communications, smart health cards and telemedicine. There will be very substantial developments in the mathematics for studying large databases. Such an approach will circumvent the current major limitation of randomised controlled trials.

In general few randomised controlled trials have been undertaken with regard to surgical or other interventions, such as coronary artery bypass surgery and percutaneous transluminal angiography (PTCA) or the subsequent insertion of a stent. Indeed few randomised controlled trials have taken place in surgery as a whole. For coronary artery bypass surgery there have been three such studies but these were undertaken many years ago and before many of the newer medical treatments were available. In the future surgical interventions and interventions with technical developments will be subjected to the same strict criteria as those which apply for drugs. It will be also necessary to follow up these trials with observational data of sufficient magnitude to have some reassurance that the benefit continues as medical practice alters with time. Some of the expertise developed in the social sciences and behavioural sciences will be needed in order to undertake such studies.

Implementation

There is little point in the detection of disease, the stratification of risk and the promotion of change in behaviour or use of a drug if there is a failure ultimately of the implementation of the medical advice. Many patients are reluctant to take medicines. Some patients dislike doctors and certainly dislike the caricature of doctors from the past to whom the pejorative phrase "doctor knows best" is applied. If the breakdown of human relations implied in such a phrase is ignored then it is probably true that a doctor does know more about the situation than the patient but that does not obviate the need to inform and speak to patients and allow patients reasonable participation in the choice of different treatments. Patients should be informed where their choice is clearly contrary to standard medical practice. Implementation of treatment in cardiovascular disease will require the co-operation of many groups not only doctors, nurses and health workers. But above all the implementation of treatments and preventive measures needs the confidence of the public and individual patients.

Delivery of health care: how and by whom?

At the present time doctors are taught medicine over a period of 5 or 6 years at medical school, then undergo a period of observation, pass subsequent examinations and finally become independent practitioners, physicians or specialists. This process is expensive and often doctors then undertake activities which do not require the extensive training which has been undertaken and financed. In cardiovascular medicine nurses are already performing minor surgery and parts of the procedure of cardiac catheterisation. The use of trained staff to undertake specific procedures will develop greatly and the number of doctors necessary to deliver technical care will fall. This will lead to considerable unhappiness and distress within the medical profession. The training programmes of doctors will be adapted to the ultimate position and needs of that individual doctor. This will require decisions to be made throughout training on the ultimate role of a doctor.

Health politics applied to cardiovascular medicine

The treatment and management of cardiovascular disease cannot be separated from the overall objective of improving health care within the population. The debate will and should be about priorities. In judging any proposed initiative the three major issues will be the traditional triad of efficacy, safety and cost. In recent years it has become commonplace for there to be a requirement that major research trials of new treatments are used as a test bed to evaluate the costs if the trial shows anticipated beneficial effects. Good examples of this problem in cardiology have been the use of ACE inhibitors for heart failure and the use of statins to lower cholesterol. Efficacy has unquestionably been shown in specific and quite broad groups of patients. Safety is largely established and where there are complications they are well known. The cost inevitably increases as less ill patients are treated because the overall benefit in such groups of patients is less. True costs are often concealed. For example a treatment which should prolong life by 2 to 3 years cannot be judged in terms of cost against older treatments with a lower mortality, a lower quality of life or an increased number of hospitalisations. An increase in duration of life can cost the community as a whole substantial sums of money, particularly if this occurs in the elderly. Patients will then develop other medical entities for which treatments will be needed and may require housing, supervision, and a pension. This total sum is the true cost. The estimation of the cost is a mathematical and scientific procedure and should not be confused or muddled with any moral decision making which may then ensue after the numbers become available. Put crudely a dead person does not result in costs to the community whereas a living person whether they be healthy or not does incur costs. The overall approach to health economics has become very confused. Some recent evidence does suggest that even if advances were to prolong life and particularly in the elderly, the costs associated would be less than the current cost of many treatments because of the smaller requirement for hospitalisation.

It is apparent that much discussion in the area of cardiovascular disease is going to be in relation to diseases of the elderly, notably coronary heart disease, heart failure, and stroke. The public expectation is for the highest quality of treatment for all. The reality will almost inevitably be that such a magnificent target is not achieved. Inevitably the pressures within society do result in particular groups of persons gaining an advantage. Public expectation will need to be broadly satisfied.

Research has resulted in very major advances in health care in the last 40 years. That has led to a widely held belief that most medical problems can be resolved by further research and it is only a lack of money which inhibits the ingenuity of man to resolve a clinical problem. That is only partly true. Advances in medicine are dependent on advances in other specialities and particularly at the present time of biology, engineering, and information technology. Much clinical research and basic scientific research is now funded by the drug industry where the business ethic is pervasive and has demonstrably been effective. A similar approach is being introduced into certain forms of research with regard to the delivery of health care and the evaluation of surgical and interventional

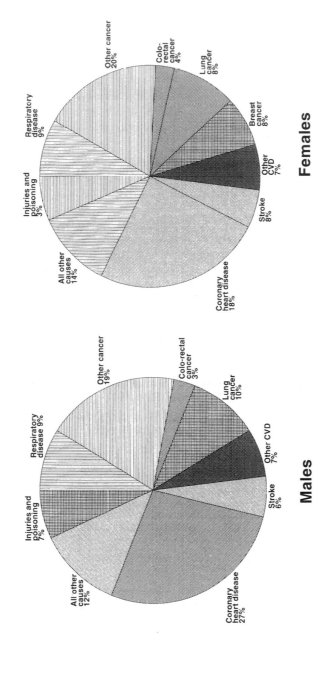

Figure 6.7   Death by cause in those under 75 years in the UK for 1995: 258 004 from a total of 641 712.

techniques. Undoubtedly this trend will accelerate and health authorities will require much harder evidence before expending large sums of public resources. The same approach is intruding into university-based research. In certain areas of science and to a limited degree it may be beneficial. The harm is that such an approach tends to snuff out innovation, and research which is unusual or unconventional ceases to get support. The universities need to and will develop programmes of research specifically directed towards innovation and the pursuance of unusual ideas. Large research groupings may be necessary in order to provide the spread of techniques often required for major research initiatives. However that very same structure can contain the seeds of destruction of output unless care is taken to nurture that which is unconventional.

Doctors are often criticised for not explaining to patients and in sufficient detail the advantages and disadvantages of particular treatments. The patient may consider themselves to be within a medical factory. That situation usually means that there is a breakdown in the relationship between doctors, health workers and the patient, although some individual patients may make it very difficult for anyone to advise them correctly even if they are making totally unreasonable decisions. This problem may partly be resolved by new methods for the transmission of information including the internet. The human problem will always remain. Doctors just like other specialists are highly trained and usually rather knowledgeable in their subject. That is why patients go to them just as they would go to a lawyer or an architect for a particular purpose. There will develop much more specific systems for handling this problem and for seeking second opinions. That does occur at present but it is in general unusual.

Medicine and law do not mix well. Breakdowns in the relationship between doctors and patients increasingly result in the involvement of the law in order to make judgements with regard to compensation. The motives of patients, lawyers and even doctors are many and various. Some are well intended, others mischievous and regrettably some promoted by greed, revenge or belligerency. Governments and society have not resolved this issue satisfactorily in any country. In the next decade new systems will be introduced taking account of the need for fairness to patients and health workers involved in these situations. These structures will allow resolution of most disputes without recourse to the full legal process as currently occurs.

A further area of change will occur in regard to the media and journals. Science and medicine suffer greatly at present from the inability of many journalists to discuss scientific issues clearly and precisely with the public. That is often because journalists do not have a scientific background and do not themselves fully understand the issues. Occasionally journalists underestimate the intelligence of their audience and trivialise issues by paraphrasing what a scientist meant to say and often says more clearly. The media have a very major role to play in altering attitudes towards health care, making society more conscious of the true costs of health decisions and encouraging individual responsibility. The provision of more information through the media will be accompanied by vast quantities of information which will be freely available on the internet.

The final consideration is the consequence of international and intercontinental action. Coronary heart disease, in particular, is a global problem. It will be the major health problem over the next 20 years both for developed and developing countries. Programmes aimed at basic research, prevention and clinical treatment will be common to many countries and continents. There will be major differences observed in relation to the consequence of certain risk factors controlled by genetics, environment and local cultures. For this reason there will be substantial growth in international cooperation in regard to the progress of research of all types into the prevention of coronary heart disease. To some extent the world is a laboratory in which natural differences between cultures and countries can be used to unravel the secrets of the origin of this wretched disorder which is causing and will cause so much human distress in the next 50 years.

Further reading

Atlas of mortality in Europe. Subnational patterns 1980/1 and 1990/1. WHO Regional Publications European Series no 75. Geneva: WHO, 1997.

Coronary heart disease statistics, 1997 edn. London: British Heart Foundation, 1997.

Murray JL, Lopez AD. Evidence-based health policy – lessons from the Global Burden of Disease Study. *Science* 1996; **274**: 740–3.

Pyorala, K, De Backer G, Graham I, Poole-Wilson PA, Wood D, on behalf of the Task Force. Prevention of coronary heart disease in clinical practice. Recommendations of the Task Force of the

European Society of Cardiology, European Atherosclerosis Society and European Society of Hypertension. *Eur Heart J* 1994; **15**: 1300–31.

References

1 Murray JL, Lopez AD. Alternative projections of mortality and disability by cause 1990–2020: Global Burden of Disease Study. *Lancet* 1997; **349**: 1498–504.
2 Tunstall-Pedoc. *Lancet* 1998; **351**: 1425–7.
3 Kelly DT. Our future society. A global challenge. *Circulation* 1997; **95**: 2459–64.
4 Department of Health, Technical Supplement, 1996. London: Department of Health.

7 Fetal and child development

Catherine Peckham

Introduction

"Clinical futures" is an amalgam of speculations, guesses and estimates by people who have expertise in an aspect of the broad field of activity on which they are commenting. Because expert opinion is plentiful, virtually inexhaustible and rarely concordant, the seriousness and wisdom of such an exercise is questionable. However, people in general, and decision-makers in particular, actually do put weight on the uncertain opinions of experts. Informed conjecture is useful if it alerts us to opportunities, threats and choices that we might not otherwise have thought about.

So in this chapter we speculate on the potential impact of some of the new clinical technologies relevant to child health within the future social context of pregnancy and childhood. Social, political and economic forces operating not only within individual communities and countries but also at a global level will shape this future. These forces, and the response to them, will influence the provision of new technologies and will require a much greater degree of public involvement in defining and making choices.

A global perspective

Centuries separate the lives and fates of children living today in different parts of the globe. The contrasts are stark and are measurable at every level, affecting all aspects of life. Foreign debt cripples parts of Africa, Asia, and Latin America. It is estimated that if African countries did not have to pay foreign creditors, the money released would save the lives of more than 20 million children by the year 2000 and provide 90 million girls and women with access to basic education. The futures, clinical and otherwise, are bleak for children living in these countries, where basic human needs such as water, food, shelter and education are poorly provided or non-existent.

There are few grounds for optimism. Future technological developments will be geared towards the needs of industrialised and emerging economies, with poor countries losing out. There are many instances of benefits which are unequally distributed between poorer and richer countries. A current and specific example is the lack of access to antiretroviral therapy for children who are infected with the HIV virus in Africa, although these children represent 80% of those affected globally. Similarly, the emergence of what has been called "information capitalism" highlights the discrepancy between individuals who have and those who do not have the skills required for using information systems and the internet for commercial and other purposes. This will induce a widening gulf between societies that are able to exploit these technologies and those that are unable to do so. As a result, social and economic inequalities will be exacerbated and there will be an inevitable increase in crime, drug addiction, child labour, child prostitution, trade in children and commerce in human spare parts, which will have serious global as well as local consequences for health.

Ironically, as the developed world moves to protect the health of its population by introducing policies, for example to reduce smoking, the hungry global market seeks out new territories and threatens the health of individuals in developing countries. As smoking declines in Europe and North America, rates are increasing in developing countries at 3% per year. If current trends persist, it is estimated that 7 million people from developing countries will die every year from smoking-related diseases. Already lung cancer in China has been increasing at the rate of 4·5% per year. Cigarette smoking is an addiction that begins in childhood and adolescence and children are the vulnerable targets of the marketing campaigns promulgated by this multinational industry.

The clinical futures evoked in this chapter relate to technologies accessible to the developed world. We gaze into the global future through a distorting glass, the distortions imposed by economic inequality in priorities and provision.

The changing demographic structure of society

In many industrialised countries both fertility and family size have declined. In Europe the fertility rate is now below that required to replace the population. As a consequence the proportion of the whole population constituted by children is falling. In the UK children comprised 25% of the population in 1960 and 19·4% in 1996. The health and welfare of children has been peripheral to the concerns of the adult population with the focus in most developed countries being on the elderly. Thus, in the health and life sciences report from the UK Office of Science and Technology Foresight Exercise, children were not mentioned at all and ageing, degenerative disease and non-specific age-related cognitive decline were identified as priorities. This emphasis will need to change as society realises the importance of investing in children and their optimal development as a means of assuring stability, prosperity, competitiveness, and cultural vigour.

The drive for this shift of emphasis is clear as the next few decades will see a progressive reduction in the proportion of people in paid employment. In Britain in 1996 there were four people of working age for every pensioner, and by 2040 there will be two. As a consequence of these demographic changes, children will be valued more as the source from which society is replenished and continuously refreshed. The preparation for meeting the responsibility of supporting ageing families and for sustaining society economically will start *in utero* and continue through carefully designed approaches to early development and upbringing.

In the UK, marked changes in family structure will continue, reflecting single and serial parenting, smaller family size, changing gender roles and changing expectations, with deferral of pregnancy until the late thirties and early forties by some women and conception in the early teenage years by others. The number of children experiencing serial parents with an extended half sibling and stepsibling network will continue to grow as a consequence of divorce. There will be a challenge to provide support for lone and often isolated parents who lack an extended family and community structure. Similarly, planning for housing, education, transport, policing and green space will need to enhance opportunities for children to interact with each other.

Social, economic and environmental influences

In developed countries the gradient in child health that exists in relation to income and social status is becoming steeper. In the UK there has been both an absolute and relative lowering of economic well-being for children in low income households and stark recognition that the relative position of children and families in society is a powerful determinant of death and ill health. The influence of socioeconomic status on child health and development must not only be acknowledged but addressed efficiently. Political solutions outside the domain of health and related services will be sought but will be difficult to achieve without rigorous analysis of the issues and incisive problem solving. Health professionals will develop a powerful advocacy role for child health, a role that is currently weak and disjointed. Ways in which, for example, education, transport, food and fiscal policies influence child health positively or negatively will be clarified and used as yardsticks to judge the validity of proposed political solutions. Social interventions such as preschool education and parent support groups will be more firmly evidence based and their future evolution shaped by the prospective testing of models informed by social, biological and other relevant knowledge.

The impact on health of the physical environment – urban and rural – will dominate policies and criteria for planning, particularly for children and adolescents for whom injury is a leading cause of death and acquired disability. The influence of both the macro- and micro-environments will be tackled together and the nature and context of impacts at different stages in a child's development elucidated. This will form the basis for preventive strategies. For example, preventive interventions for childhood asthma will be based on an understanding of the relative contributions of the macro-environment (e.g., traffic fumes, air pollution) and the micro-environment (e.g., house dust mite, passive smoking, gas cooking, damp housing).

The impact of lifestyle and behaviour

Many adult lifestyles, relating for example to dietary patterns, physical activity and risk-taking behaviour, are laid down in childhood and adolescence. Because of the changes in social patterns within families, healthy lifestyles will be more difficult to maintain in the future. Passive entertainment such as television viewing and computer games, physical inactivity and meals as isolated rather than social events, will enhance risk factors for disease in adult life and result in a downward shift in the age at onset of conditions such as osteoporosis and cardiovascular disease. This trend will place demands on health services and offset the benefits that may have accrued from other lifestyle changes, such as a reduction in smoking. Rather than changing lifestyle, there will be an increasing medicalisation of high-risk groups designed to prevent the consequences of an unhealthy lifestyle. There will be increased reliance on pills rather than exercise for osteoporosis, on antidepressants instead of social support for depression, and on usage of cholesterol-lowering drugs in later life instead of dietary change. There will be a continued reduction in the age at first sexual intercourse, particularly for girls, with consequences for sexually transmitted disease, teenage pregnancy and risks of involuntary infertility in later life. Drug use, both legal and illegal, will rise leading to increasing addiction among the young.

Changing patterns of childhood morbidity

With the development of new vaccines and a reduction in infectious diseases, the major burden of childhood disease will be due to chronic conditions such as asthma, diabetes and disability, particularly that arising from the increasing survival of very premature infants. Cure rates from childhood cancer will continue to improve and children with conditions such as cystic fibrosis will have an extended lifespan. However, at the same time there will be a rise in problems reflecting lifestyle and other issues, including obesity, anorexia, and behavioural disorders. We are only just beginning to address the influence this may have for adults.

Novel and non-invasive routes of vaccine administration will be used, such as genetically modified food or aerosols, and new and effective combination vaccines will be available for a wider number of infections ranging from HIV to otitis media. Immunisation will continue to have a huge impact in reducing the mortality and morbidity associated with childhood infections and polio will have been eradicated globally. However, adults will require repeated vaccination into old age in order to maintain adequate levels of immunity throughout life. Paradoxically, despite the declining incidence of infectious disease, high vaccination levels will be difficult to maintain as belief in the need for "herd" immunity becomes dominated by individual concerns. A growing group of parents, with no personal experience of the infectious diseases vaccines aim to prevent, will not perceive the need to continue to have their child protected and the focus will be on the potential harm of immunisation. Onset of childhood conditions which are temporally associated with immunisation will fuel the deep rooted belief that immunisation causes all kinds of health problems and damages the immune system. New outbreaks of "old diseases" such as rubella will happen, as a result of declining immunity and increased travel to areas where these diseases are still prevalent, leading to, for example, the birth of infants with congenital rubella. At the same time, there will be ongoing debate as to when and to whom the new vaccines, for example against cancer, should be given. Antibiotic drug resistance, with fewer antibiotics available for treatment of childhood infections, will stimulate vaccine development.

The adult as a grown-up child: early determinants of future disease

Much of what is said in this chapter concentrates on features of fetal life and childhood, which are precursors of health and ill health in adults. Factors that influence health may operate independently at an early stage of development or in the young child, or interact with influences that continue throughout adolescence into adult life. An increasing and substantial number of adults will have received treatment for a childhood condition that was previously fatal. At present about 1 in 1000 adults in the UK are survivors of childhood cancer and this proportion will grow. Children surviving neonatal intensive care, better management of previously lethal inherited conditions such as cystic fibrosis, and successful treatment for congenital anomalies will add to this pool. In some cases this will have a direct impact on adult medicine and health-care resources, for example through longer survival from chronic disease. In other cases there may be undetected – possibly genetic – sequelae which will add in the short or longer term to adult burdens of ill health.

Longitudinal studies will elucidate the causal pathways that link early life, childhood development, and adult health status. For some conditions, such as diabetes and heart and lung disease, these pathways will be traced back to factors operating in fetal life including the intrauterine environment. The effects of continuity of exposure through life to factors that influence the intrauterine environment and that also influence childhood development and adult disease will be clarified. For example, low weight at birth, which is itself a marker of socioeconomic status, is associated with continuing socioeconomic disadvantage throughout childhood and adolescence. The complex biological and social mechanisms that result in low weight at birth will be understood and this will lead to the design of effective preventive interventions.

There will be firm evidence that juvenile delinquency and adult criminal activity can be predicted in early life and that its cause is largely due to poor parenting and deprived backgrounds. There will be accumulating evidence to show that interventions to mitigate or avoid the intergenerational consequences of poor parenting for vulnerable children are successful and highly cost effective.

Pregnancy and childbirth

The risk of pathology before or after birth is set, to an unknown extent, by the genetic constitution of the mother and the father and the genes inherited by the child. The expression of risk is modulated by environmental factors *in utero* and postnatally, through to adult life and old age. The genetic constitution of the mother and father interacting with external factors will shape the child's development postnatally into adolescence and beyond.

In general, scientists will continue to find it easier and more attractive to tackle genetic rather than environmental questions. However, there will be public and political pressure to identify effective secondary preventive interventions, thereby giving more priority to characterising gene–environment interactions. The influence of maternal genetic and non-genetic factors on the milieu of pregnancy, operating, for example, through placental function as well as through external influences such as food intake, alcohol and smoking, will be clarified.

As these influences are better understood there will be increased emphasis on pre-fertilisation parental fitness, with women offered screening for factors likely to affect the future fetus, such as genotype, infection, and nutrition. Uterus transplants will be available for women who require them. The prevention, postponement or attenuation of adult disease and the modulation of ageing processes will be sought through early interventions. This will lead to pressure for preconception and preimplantation screening. There may also be increased demand for gender selection. By cloning sections of DNA that code for physical or mental features, genetic engineering will have the potential to produce designer babies, but only for those that can afford it. As genetic risk is better understood there will be pressure for interventions where the DNA from somatic cells of genetically "clean" or "desirable" sources will be used to fertilise ova also from carefully selected sources. This will raise issues of discrimination, morality, ethics, and public acceptance.

Wider ranging genetic screening based on the recovery of fetal cells from maternal blood will be undertaken to determine fetal genotype. The majority of gene defects resulting in childhood disorders and other inherited conditions will be detectable, but identification of genes in the conceptus or fetus, such as the *BRCA* mutations, which may increase susceptibility to disease in adult life, through interaction with environmental factors, will lead to action without adequate knowledge.

This will have implications for primary prevention through preimplantation diagnosis as well as for secondary prevention through termination of pregnancy and *in utero* gene therapy. The feasibility of preventing fetal abnormalities and genetically inherited disorders will challenge society to retain a pluralistic approach where individual choice is respected and supported. Alternatively, parents who proceed with a pregnancy in the knowledge that their fetus is handicapped or at very high risk of a disorder, such as Down syndrome, cystic fibrosis or a severe congenital abnormality, may be stigmatised by society and expected to meet the costs of care and treatment. At the same time, failure to detect affected pregnancies through established screening programmes will raise the prospect of legal actions by children against their parents, the state, or those responsible for "intra-uterine health care".

The expectation will be that women should have healthy babies with everything done to minimise risk to the fetus and newborn, bearing in mind that most babies are born healthy with the minimum amount of medical intervention and that most women want reassurance that their baby is normal. User-friendly methods of monitoring fetal development will be devised for pregnant women to use at home. The images and information so generated will be relayed digitally by telephone to a central service where automated assessment using preset criteria will be used to alert professionals and the pregnant woman to the need for review. Such measures will lead to the compilation of a large body of longitudinal data contributing to a better understanding of intrauterine growth and development.

Women will continue to want to have their babies delivered by friendly, professionally capable staff in a non-threatening environment. Few women will seek home births as a positive option and it seems unlikely, at least in Britain, that there will be an increased demand for home deliveries over the coming decades. Instead, emphasis will be placed on providing a homely environment in hospital where the woman feels in control and has rapid access to expert obstetric or paediatric facilities if required.

Health and development *in utero* and in childhood: a new focus for medicine

Health and development *in utero* and in the early childhood years will emerge as the central focus of medicine, as the genesis of adult disease and ageing is understood and the possibilities of influencing physical, medical and social development are recognised and exploited. There will be a tension between the application of technology to achieve the perfect individual and its use to understand how environmental changes may be used to maximise the potential of individuals as they are.

There will be major advances in functional imaging techniques to detect structural abnormalities and in the assessment of fetal organ function. Imaging technology will substitute completely for invasive diagnosis. Three-dimensional ultrasonographic, echo-cardiographic and magnetic resonance imaging will become the gold standard for the next generation, not only to make accurate anatomical diagnosis but also to provide detailed functional assessments before, during and after therapeutic interventions. Very fast acquisition sequences for magnetic resonance imaging will be available and will be exploited to image the fetus. Most anatomical abnormalities of the fetus will be detected in the first half of pregnancy, even those that are relatively subtle and effectively treated, such as cleft palate or talipes.

Brain function will be assessed through qualitative assessment of neuronal migration, synaptogenesis, and cerebral biochemical function. Additional insights will be provided by magnetic resonance and/or near infrared spectroscopy with magnetic stimulation of developing neural pathways being used to assess the developing motor system of the early fetus. Non-invasive, probably transcutaneous methods, will be used to monitor the health of babies *in utero* through the mother's abdominal wall. Fetal well-being will also be assessed through measurement of acid balance, blood gases, cardiovascular function, and metabolic state.

A range of interventions will be developed, including technologically based ways of influencing fetal growth and development, for example through modifying placental function and modulating nutrition *in utero*. More effective methods to support the compromised fetus into the third trimester of pregnancy will be available to allow for safe delivery of the premature newborn infant.

Twins and multiple births expose the babies to a significantly increased risk of handicap. As there is no biological advantage to being a twin, improved methods will be developed for reducing the number of multiple pregnancies. Multiple births as a result of infertility treatment are already being discouraged, and it is probable that multiple birth as a result of any form of infertility treatment will become unacceptable. This will raise the issue of selective termination of a co-twin early in pregnancy for those multiple births occurring spontaneously. The ethics of this will be more widely discussed in view of the doubling of risk of disability to a twin pair.

Although early and accurate assessment of organ function will be possible in the first trimester it is unlikely that fetal surgery will prove effective at this stage. Termination of pregnancy will therefore remain the only therapeutic option. However, detection of abnormalities in the second trimester will open the way for fetal surgery. Fetal organ transplantation will become an effective and feasible form of therapy for all major systems, but this will not be necessary in the majority of cases until near, or at the time, of delivery. Rather than planning an intervention during pregnancy, early detection with delivery in the appropriate surgical/transplantation environment will be necessary. In the early 1980s, the introduction of intrauterine echocardiographic diagnosis of congenital heart disease led to the termination of fetuses with highly correctable congenital malformations, a trend that was reversed in the early 1990s. The decision to terminate or operate will be clearer, as more refined assessments of congenital heart disease in the fetus will be available together with information on the long term results of repaired congenital heart disease.

Ethical dilemmas relating to the concept of the "perfect fetus" will be revisited, with tensions between the rights of the fetus, the mother and society to determine the fate of affected pregnancies where the fetal abnormality is compatible with life, and treatable but not curable. The combination of improved fetal surveillance, enhanced expectations of a normal child and the ready acceptance of termination will make ethical decisions difficult, particularly for minor or treatable abnormalities or for those of uncertain outcome.

Prematurity

There are many reasons for premature birth which need to be considered separately in order to understand whether prevention is desirable or feasible. At present 7% of babies born in the UK are premature (<37 completed weeks of pregnancy) and 1% are severely premature (birthweight <1500 g or gestation <30 weeks). These proportions will not decline and may well increase, with a greater proportion born severely premature. This increase will be mainly due to iatrogenic premature delivery of women not in labour.

Where chronic or sporadic maternal conditions predispose women to recurrent premature delivery, the fetus is probably healthy and suppression of prematurity is appropriate. More effective treatment will be available to suppress premature labour. Maternal infections will continue to trigger early onset of labour. Although screening will be in place and there will be more effective antimicrobials, antibiotic resistance will become a major problem. However, vaccines against important pathogens such as streptococcus B will become increasingly available.

Babies who fail to thrive *in utero* will be delivered in a very premature state as technological advances will ensure that the premature delivery of a severely compromised fetus offers a higher chance of survival in the neonatal intensive care unit than in the uterus. However, this practice will have profound implications for the quality of life of survivors and their families. Some women will suffer multiple miscarriage or very early onset of premature labour despite treatment. For those women with an apparently healthy conceptus, an artificial womb will become a reality. Within 10 years it will be possible to transplant a viable immature fetus from the mother into an artificial environment which will nurture the pregnancy to a point where safe delivery can occur. Factors that will inhibit this from happening are ethical and financial. Although it will be difficult to reconcile the costs and benefits of this form of treatment, which will be appropriate for perhaps only 0·1% of fertile women, the pressure of potential beneficiaries supported by the media will be emotive and persuasive.

Consequences of premature birth

Currently approximately 10% of babies born very prematurely survive with some disability, of which 5% will be severely disabled. A further 20–30% of very immature babies who survive will have disabilities with no "hard" neurological signs. These disabilities include clumsiness, attention deficit disorder, poor school performance, and mild to moderate learning problems. These problems will not feature in the neonatal period, where questions of life, death and severe handicap are to the fore, but will emerge later when such "minor" disabilities will cause major problems in school and at home.

The full range of long-term psychological sequelae of extreme prematurity are only now beginning to be appreciated. Understanding of the mechanisms underlying the psychological development of very premature infants will have accumulated and this will be used to devise successful preventive strategies. There are 50–60 times more extremely low birth weight (< 1000 g) children surviving now compared with the early 1960s. The impact of this on the community will be substantial, as the prevalence of psychological deficits will be substantially greater although levels of disability in this group will have declined.

The increased risk of severe disability in premature infants will be predicted by methods for assessing the developing brain. Both motor and cognitive function, and hearing and vision will be assessed in the first few days after birth. It will be possible to make an accurate prognosis of a very high risk of poor outcome due to acquired brain damage. If a critical amount of brain damage has been sustained, it is unlikely that this will prove treatable. Prognosis, based on these techniques, might inform withdrawal of life support and, in some instances, the case for active euthanasia will be strongly argued.

Acquired damage to the developing brain due to prematurity, birth injury, or asphyxia, will be treated to prevent, or ameliorate, functional brain damage. High-risk babies will be treated prior to premature delivery by medication administered to the mother. These medicines will have a range of actions designed to stabilise cerebral blood flow, reduce coagulation disturbances, and minimise free radical injury. Effective intervention therapies in babies with established brain injury will also be developed. Brain hypothermia is promising but safety issues need to be resolved. It may well be used for acute brain injury in older children and adults. However, it is unlikely that there will be one therapy that achieves neuroprotection through all the possible pathways, and a combination of pharmaceutical and technological interventions will be used.

A number of strategies will be developed to understand the

causes of disabilities in premature infants and to reduce their incidence. The approaches will be either interventional or enhancement related. The causes of less severe neurological disability are many, but nutrition is likely to play an important role. Human-based milk formulas will be adapted to the needs of prematurely born infants and will be based on recombinant DNA technology so that the fat and protein will be human rather than cow or vegetable. More appropriate nutrition (both milk based and parenteral) will reduce neuronal dropout as a result of premature birth. Anti-oxidants, such as vitamin E, will be given to reduce cytokine-induced neuronal damage, either during pregnancy to women at high risk of premature delivery, or to the premature baby.

Enhancement therapy will be directed towards providing an appropriately enriched environment for children at risk of developmental problems. Special programmes will be designed to provide the requisite stimulation for encouraging the relatively "plastic" immature brain to compensate for damaged areas. These therapies, provided by a new cadre of generic teachers with advanced therapy skills, will also be valuable for children from deprived backgrounds who will benefit from focused stimulation. These programmes will start at, or shortly after, birth and continue for the first few years before dovetailing into mainline schooling.

Paediatric surgical issues: the example of congenital heart disease

> It will make a nice bedtime story for my great-grandchildren to tell them that one of their ancestors spent his life tying knots inside the hearts of small babies

Basic surgical techniques such as the use of threads to approximate anatomic structures will be relegated to history books as sealing agents replace sewing procedures. With optical technology, it will be possible to see through blood and to repair some cardiovascular defects using endovascular devices without opening the heart or the great vessels. Video-assisted technology and telesurgery will make it possible to operate from a distance and greater precision and accuracy of surgical repairs will be achieved. Patients will have the choice between a machine-made or a handmade repair of their heart defect. Minimally invasive cardiac surgery, currently only used in adults, will be undertaken in children.

Experimentation with alternative methods of providing extracorporeal circulation will feature, although cardiopulmonary bypass will remain necessary for some surgical procedures. The cascade of events leading to tissue and cellular injury following cardiopulmonary bypass will be understood and lead to novel approaches to prevent and/or treat the side effects of this procedure. Transgenic blood, blood substitutes and prepared blood that is safe will provide blood devoid of human risk factors. The risk of transmitting viruses from animal donors will remain a concern.

Cardiac substitutes

Although there will be complete tolerance of transplanted human organs, their use will be limited because of shortage of donors. Xenotransplantation and organ cloning will be used to provide alternative sources of organs. The development of transgenic animals will make xenotransplantation feasible, but the problem of possible viral contamination of the recipient and, more importantly, of the human species, will restrict their use. Cloning of spare parts, for example a spare heart from fetal cells, will enable transplants to be carried out at birth or even before, using the maternal placenta as a natural "heart lung machine". Pending the discovery of biocompatible and non-thrombogenic material and of implantable long-lasting power sources, artificial mechanical hearts may become an alternative.

Genetic and molecular therapies

Current research in molecular and genetic engineering will produce a wealth of potential therapeutic opportunities. Developments in gene therapy will include the rapid induction of cell hypertrophy, for example to prepare a low pressure ventricle to serve the systemic circulation; the induction of proteins that facilitate recovery from ischaemic injury following repair of complex cardiac defects; and the induction of new myocyte growth, for example around an extracardiac conduit, to support the Fontan circulation. Rational drug design with enhanced target specificity will lead to the development of drugs acting on specific cells, such as lymphatic myocytes. This will be a major advance in the treatment of conditions that have in common interstitial oedema and effusions, such as congestive heart failure or the failing Fontan circulation.

Health care for children

As a group, children will continue to make low demands on the acute health-care system with a small proportion of severely ill children requiring specialist and intensive "high tech" medicine. The last century's iatrogenic epidemics of tonsillectomy and grommet insertion will be replaced by the medicalisation of children with societal diseases such as obesity, anorexia, hyperactivity, and attention deficit disorders, as well as addictions to tobacco, alcohol and other drugs.

Paediatric care will be further dichotomised between community-based and highly specialised care. Most sick children will not be seen in hospital and appropriate care will be given at home or in clinics close by. Hospital care will be reserved for those critically ill children who cannot be looked after safely in these settings. As a result, children's hospitals will become fewer in number, each providing care for a population of about 5 million people. Hospital services will revolve around the intensive care unit dealing with acute life threatening illness and trauma, supported by an appropriate concentration of specialised medical, nursing and other skills. The care of critically ill children will be greatly enhanced by advances in the non-invasive monitoring of organ systems. The need for invasive procedures will be minimised or avoided and more effective methods will be available for supporting the heart and respiratory systems. Respiratory failure will remain the major reason for children requiring intensive care. The role and the status of nurses and other key non-medical staff in highly specialised areas of practice will be acknowledged and upgraded to reflect their knowledge, expertise and responsibilities. A single hierarchy will emerge, with nurses and doctors occupying positions commensurate with their expertise and responsibilities.

Thus, there will be a progressive shift towards child health primary care for disease prevention and the management of acute and chronic illness and disability. The creation of large primary care consortia will lead to community-based medical subspecialisation with the disappearance of the general medical practitioner. Nurses and other non-medical staff will take on a range of specialised roles within primary care, but will also assume the generalist mantle. Case management advice and the monitoring of treatment and follow-up will be aided by telemedicine linkages within primary care, between patients and primary care, between primary care centres and hospitals and between hospitals. International transfer of information will become routine to aid the diagnosis and treatment of complex and rare problems. This will become a major route through which the expertise and facilities of the richer countries can be shared with the developing world.

Economic criteria will dominate policy decisions about the future of expensive high technology health care. High technology medicine will be performed exclusively in units, with a critical mass of patients supported by a team of highly specialised experts who will also play a role in research and development, as well as the training and education of future experts. What constitutes critical mass in terms of number of patients, number and diversity of staff and facilities, will be based on comparative economic and outcomes data, taking geographical location, population density and requirement for specialised care into account. The increased cost of the NHS will be such that care will become increasingly divorced from diagnosis, treatment and high technology procedures. Parents will become increasingly disenchanted with the failure of technology to live up to its expectation. The use of complementary medicine will gain widespread public acceptance. The new challenge will be to ensure that complementary medicines are fully integrated with orthodox medicine to enhance quality of life, while respecting the principles of scientific evaluation.

Outcomes-related accountability will provide the basis for liability and there will be an exponential rise in legal actions against surgeons in general, and paediatric cardiac surgeons in particular. Appropriate mechanisms for providing compensation against non-negligent harm resulting from medical and/or surgical interventions will be in place in some regions. Failures in high technology medicine – a hallmark of complex sociotechnical systems – will be examined as failures of a system as well as of an individual.

However, the changed pattern of delivery of orthodox health care to children will not address the roots of childhood health problems and community solutions will be sought. Unless they take on a child advocacy role, child health professionals may find themselves increasingly isolated, with society demanding more in relation to its children. Individuals will be identified from within communities to take responsibility for community issues such as teenage pregnancy. Cooperative health groups will be set up. Health visitors will be reinstated and work to identify vulnerable children at a stage when early intervention will have the greatest benefit. The school health service will re-emerge with a strengthened remit to support and promote lifestyle and behavioural practices compatible with longevity and reduced morbidity.

Future scenarios

New knowledge regarding the influence of psychosocial and socioeconomic factors and brain development will generate political controversy over the coming decades. Evidence of the importance of early childhood development as a lifelong determinant of health, well-being, and competence will threaten contemporary notions of family privacy and autonomy. This in turn will induce a protective reaction in favour of the exclusive right of the family to bring up children as it sees fit. At the same time, there will be a heightened sense of urgency to take collective responsibility for the early childhood years. The political left will focus on the equitable distribution of opportunities and the right will give emphasis to producing a cognitively sophisticated population which can "compete" in the global economy. These latent conflicts and tensions evoke a number of possible future scenarios. Two are presented: one we would like to see and the other we are afraid we will see.

The preferred scenario

Fifty years from now, there will be broad acceptance of the fundamental importance of nature–nurture interactions and arguments of a "nature versus nurture" debate will seem as crude and as sinister to us then as turn-of-the-century eugenics concepts do to us today. The scientific basis of this scenario will be a thorough understanding of the role of critical and sensitive periods in human brain development during the first 5 years of life. The crucial elements will be scientific consensus on "how critical is critical" and "how sensitive is sensitive?" In other words, to what extent windows of opportunity for the development of specific competencies in the brain "open" only once, and for circumscribed periods of time, and to what extent they can be stretched, re-opened, or efficiently replaced by alternative pathways which open in later life. This knowledge will be complemented by scientific development in two other areas.

First, outstanding issues surrounding the presence or absence of hierarchies in the development of brain competencies will be settled. Most important of these will be an understanding of the extent to which high quality emotional/affiliative experiences in the first 2 years of life are a precondition for successful intellectual development thereafter. Second, the extent to which specific early experiences, operating through mechanisms that act independently or together, affect subsequent health and well-being will be understood. These mechanisms may operate through exerting an effect irrespective of intervening experience (through latency); through life pathways that are engendered by early experiences (thus shaping their environment for opportunity); and through accumulation of risk or resilience according to the intensity and duration of developmentally significant experiences.

Each effect model will be shown to make important contributions, and the hidden political arguments which currently lead investigators and policy makers to advocate only one model at the expense of others will be pre-empted by coordinated analyses of birth cohort studies, producing a consensus on the relative importance of each model. Moreover, the axes which link the developing brain to the body's host defence mechanisms will be thoroughly characterised. We will understand how, when, and to what extent the psychoneuro–endocrine and psychoneuro–immune axes of the developing human become conditioned by psychosocial and socioeconomic experiences, and the degree to which systematic differences in the disposition of these axes, according to differential life experiences, contribute to socioeconomic gradients in health status.

The scientific understanding described above will be complemented by a renewed social commitment to children. The basic principle will be summarised by the maxim "do not let any group of children be left behind". The social corollary will be a policy of universal access to the conditions of healthy child development. Seven conditions will be identified: adequate income; access to facilities, emotional and social support; intellectual stimulation; adequate nutrition; sensible/quality care arrangements; individual advocacy/mentorship by at least one socially legitimate adult; and safety (ranging from vaccination to protect from infectious diseases to protection from physical abuse and unintentional injury).

Identifying this simple set of determinants of healthy child development will be the easy part, guaranteeing each child access to them will prove much harder. Within a few decades many countries will be using population-based, person-specific, longitudinal reporting systems to monitor progress and to evaluate periodically each child's access to the seven factors. The methods used to improve access will largely be left up to communities and families in order to minimise invasion of privacy, but a system of accountability for outcomes will be established, with greater or lesser enforceability, in different jurisdictions. Decisions will be made about how to use the threat of trade restrictions under international agreement, to bring wayward countries into line.

This focus on outcome will create pressure for progress in five domains. First, through developmental, psychological and brain imaging techniques, advances will be made in understanding individual variation in the development of specific competencies. In particular, we will know a great deal more about how to open developmental pathways through, for example, exposure to music, physical activity, the use of computer methods for combating dyslexia, and the balance between phonetics and whole language approaches to reading. The one-size-fits-all approach to education will be abandoned, although doing so without compromising universal access will prove to be difficult.

A second area of progress will help solve this latter problem. The inexorable decline in demand for acute care paediatric services, due to decreasing fertility rates and lower levels of paediatric morbidity, will lead to a planned re-deployment of child health care funding towards "child developmental resource centres". These centres will carry out individual developmental assessments, using state of the art techniques, in order to help parents and schools identify an individualised educational plan for each child and to help troubleshoot and modify the plan over time. By strategically merging paediatric and educational resources in this way, the process of developing special educational plans in the context of a universal education system will be made simpler.

The other three areas of progress will complement the above, but will take effect at a broader level of social aggregation. Neighbourhood environments will be required to provide a wide range of opportunities for physical stimulation and interaction with other children, through a variety of play spaces, especially where housing is physically restrictive to young children. A "life credit" system will be available for those leaving the workplace to take on primary childcare responsibilities; and a range of social policies to smooth out work-life/home-life conflicts will be implemented. Finally, pay scales for those providing licensed child care will rise dramatically to reflect the importance of this role, and infrastructure funding for child-care centres will be improved to reflect the developmental needs of young children.

The alternative scenario

The alternative scenario, which sadly we are more likely to see, will result from the following tendencies, which if they are not held in check will undermine the efforts outlined above. The potential exists for the development of genetic screening for multifactorial conditions, whose genetic contribution, if it exists at all, exists only in interaction with environmental factors. The conjunction of genetic screening, entrepreneurial initiative, and a willingness to rush to label individuals and fetuses as being "at risk" might well undermine efforts to improve the environment for child development. This will occur directly, through spending choices, and indirectly, through the promulgation of the notion of strict genetic determinism.

Although neurobiology has the potential to sharpen our understanding of how to create optimal environments for child development, this will not be regarded as a profitable area for investment. The lion's share of resources will go primarily to drug-related research, and 50 years from now the principles of child development will be no better understood than they are today. Polarisation between those who believe the environment is the most important determinant of health and those who believe that genetic risk is more important will increase. It is likely that social inequalities relating to lifestyles and prevention will get bigger despite increasing equity of access to health services.

More likely, and more insidious, would be a scenario in which those who understand the importance of early child development use their privileged knowledge to abandon those children who are at risk of failure, so that universal access to quality education would be progressively eroded through "reforms" in education funding mechanisms. Increased knowledge of the role of early child development may also bring back a form of aggressive "nanny-ism". This would mean an increasingly punitive attitude towards those who do not provide an exemplary environment for their children, but without distinguishing between those who lack resources and those who lack commitment. In an era where adoptable children will become increasingly scarce, child confiscations might become the preferred method of enhancing living conditions for children, rather than efforts at the cross-the-board improvements described above.

Conclusions

The goals of paediatric medicine are twofold: to foster the normal health and development of the child, and to advance the prevention and treatment of childhood illness. In pursuit of these goals, it is essential to consider the social and economic nature of the society in which children live, as well as the structure, circumstances and social and economic position of their own family within that society. A child's upbringing reflects this macroenvironment, with early experiences being further modified by the parenting they receive. For children's health particularly, there is a tension between socioeconomic and cultural factors on the one hand, and scientific and technological change on the other. The growing prominence of biotechnology emphasises the divorce of the individual from the social context. As Foucault observes, medicine conceives of diseases as "abstract essences", so that to perform a "medical reading" the doctor has "to take the patient into account only to place him in parentheses". This resonates with the sentiments expressed by Margaret Lock, the anthropologist, who described the scientific view of the body as "reified, isolated, decontextualised, and abstracted from real time, actual location and social space". This view, reinforced by commercial pressures and supported by professional and scientific interests, may be strategically useful for certain aspects of medicine. However, it will be increasingly challenged, as the interdependence between biology and social environment, which is particularly expressed by a mother and her developing child, becomes better understood. Sensitivity to, and respect for, this interdependence must provide a foundation for enlightened policies and practice.

The following contributed substantial passages which are incorporated in this chapter:

Carol Dezateux
Senior Lecturer, Epidemiology and Public Health, Institute of Child Health, London, UK

Clyde Hertzman
Associate Professor of Health Care and Epidemiology, Department of Health Care and Epidemiology, University of British Columbia, Vancouver, Canada

Marc de Leval
Lead Clinician in Cardiac Surgery, Great Ormond Street Hospital,
London, UK

Malcolm Levene
Professor of Paediatrics, Division of Paediatrics and Child Health,
The General Infirmary at Leeds, Leeds, UK

8 Ageing

John Grimley Evans

Speculating about the future is a diverting if vain exercise. To the mystic the future is merely a withered rose and the cosmologist can take refuge in an infinite number of futures, but ordinary men can only look to windward. We can note the bearing of current knowledge and technology, and form some opinion about the direction and strength of social and political breezes. We can only look forward by looking back.

Retrospect

There is a common misapprehension that old age is a new phenomenon produced, in some sense artificially, by economic development, medical science, or the welfare state. In fact, old age has always been with us. In classical Greece men lived into their eighties and nineties. Sophocles lived to 91, Isocrates committed suicide at 98. Agesilaus II, King of Sparta, died in his 85th year on the way home from Egypt where he had been leading an active military campaign. Studies of hunter-gatherer societies show that 20% of individuals reached the age of 60 and 10% the age of 70.[1] The common myth that in olden times people were "old by 35" is based on a misunderstanding of life expectancy. Life expectancy is the average age at death and is heavily determined by rates of infant mortality. Survivors of childhood have always done well in terms of length of life. Indeed where infant mortality is high natural selection is at work and the survivors are correspondingly resilient. Within living memory Indian men of 50 were on average outliving British men of the same age. What has changed is not the genetically determined maximum length of human life but the environmentally determined proportion of us who achieve something near to our genetic potential for longevity.

The diseases and disabilities associated with old age have also been recognised since the earliest records. The twelfth chapter of

Ecclesiastes is an extended poetic allegory of the afflictions of later life. Hippocrates taught about them. Aristotle discourses disparagingly on the mental attributes of older men but probably mistook for the effects of age the disillusionment of cohorts of Athenians humiliated in the Peloponnesian War and the conquests of Alexander. (He may also have been oblivious of the personal animosity older Athenians felt towards him as Alexander's tutor.)

As the tragic tale of Tithonus testifies, man has long recognised his dilemma in wanting to live long but not wanting to be old. Nowadays most of us live long enough to realise that immortality would be a dubious blessing. It would threaten boredom and the endless disappointment of finding that things never get any better, but merely become unsatisfactory in different ways. An eternity of television soap operas appeals no more strongly to the modern man of parts than previously promised eternities of listening to hosannas ringing between the nine orders of angels. Present generations, indeed, may die with a sense of relief that they have not survived to see any of the world catastrophes that unbridled human venery, environmental depletion, international capitalism and lunatic religions seem to be making inevitable. Immortality is a minority taste, and the notion that all humanity is in pursuit of it[2] merely a health economist's fantasy.

There are cultural as well as individual differences however. English culture has inherited an indelible colouring from the Wyrd of the Anglo-Saxons, Wyrd being the ruling pattern of events to which even the gods are subject. For the English, in the words put into the mouth of Julius Caesar by Shakespeare, death is not something to be feared but "a necessary end that will come when it will come". Even the English Christians, again in Shakespeare's words, recognised themselves as "owing God a death". Sir Thomas Browne, the most English of Christians, was ashamed of death not afraid of it. But things may be changing. Beyond the Pale of Anglo-Saxon culture, in the anomic groves of California, can be found earnest believers in an indefinite lifespan as a desirable possibility within the grasp of present generations. Is this just the dream of a privileged minority or the voice of the world-future, or at least of the affluent world-future? "Birth and copulation and death" were all the facts to the generation of Apeneck Sweeney,[3] but as more people live beyond and outside the span of biological necessity perhaps we will all develop some new hopes of long life. Our old-world accidie, Weltschmerz, or boredom may be no more than means of diffusing the cognitive dissonance between innate immortal longings and the past realities of a European world too often trampled by the horsemen of the apocalypse.

Be that as it may, even if in the UK we can expect our present emphasis on quality rather than length of life to survive another generation, we shall be in earshot of alien voices bewailing their mortality. Moreover, traditional processes of acculturation in the UK are being subverted by the media and commerce. Although recognising that the Global Village may be no more enticing than Los Angeles on a smoggy December afternoon, we may face a future preoccupied with extending the duration of life at any price.

Here and now

In the UK, concern about the welfare of older people was inspired by the medical profession, and particularly by the specialty of geriatric medicine created by the NHS in 1948. This led to a degree of "medicalisation" of old age that some social scientists have found objectionable. Most older people, however, nominate good health as their primary concern, even while recognising that wealth, housing, family attachments, social integration and leisure activities are also important contributors to human happiness.

In this regard, present trends are encouraging. In the USA older people are living longer and are fitter.[4] Age-specific disability rates and needs for health care in later life are falling. The rate of growth in the numbers of older people is still outstripping these improvements so that the total volume of need for services continues to rise but less than the data of 10 or 20 years ago would have predicted. It seems likely that adoption of healthy lifestyles has made an important contribution to these promising trends. We have no idea what is happening in the UK because we do not gather the necessary information. The American data do however tell us what could be made to happen here if we have the will to provide our citizenry with the opportunities and incentives they need to adopt healthier lifestyles. Good advice and exhortatory leaflets from the Health Education Authority are not enough; they may improve knowledge but are unlikely, by themselves, to influence behaviour.

The UK also suffers from political ambivalence. Politicians and civil servants fear that medical or biological research on ageing, or even decent quality health care for older people, may have expensive implications for the NHS. It is assumed that the longer one lives the greater the burden one places on the taxpayer. This is not necessarily so but it makes all too plausible a story. There are many virtues in a socialised system of health care, but one major disadvantage is the paralysing effect on innovation as politicians toady to tactically voting taxpayers. The indifference to the fate of people aged over 65, implicit in the recent Green Paper "Our Healthier Nation", tells us clearly where the Department of Health stands.

The nature and causes of ageing

Ageing, as a biological phenomenon, is characterised by a loss of adaptability of an individual organism over time. As we grow older we lose functional reserve and become less able to resist and recover from diseases. This loss of adaptability forms the subject matter of the biological gerontologist and the challenge to the geriatrician. It is important to bear in mind however that even if we were to abolish ageing we would still all eventually die from accident, disease, famine, or warfare. Moreover, the longer we survive the more we become liable to time-dependent hazards. Time dictates the accumulation of deleterious products of genes, and the cumulative effects of imbalances in dietary intake and energy output. We are also subject to cumulative effects of environmental carcinogens such as our own or other people's tobacco smoke. The incidence of some cancers rises as a function not of age but of duration and intensity of exposure to carcinogens. The rise with age in incidence and fatality of disease is due therefore partly to ageing and partly to time. Time and age are closely linked but may not always start at the same point or march at the same pace. In most countries incidence and fatality of diseases also reflect discrimination against older people in that they are subjected to more poverty, poorer housing and lower quality health care than are other age groups. Even if ageing were prevented, therefore, we should not expect universal immortality.

Ageing is the product of extrinsic factors in environment and lifestyle interacting with intrinsic (genetic) factors. In general we will live longer if we exercise and maintain a sensible body weight. Some of us carry genes that lead to hypertension if we eat too much salt. We differ genetically in how we metabolise carcinogens in tobacco smoke. However, we all carry genes whose actions are insufficient to keep us alive for ever. Chief among these are the genes that determine the effectiveness of damage control. Our cells and bodies are being assaulted constantly by damaging influences including heat, radiation and the products of our own metabolism. Damage control mechanisms include prevention, detection, repair, and replacement. We could only survive indefinitely if these processes were 100% effective, but under conditions of natural selection they will of necessity be less than that. Damage control is expensive in energy and can only be carried out by reducing the rate of reproduction. An organism that devotes sufficient energy to damage control to abolish ageing will be outbred by competitors who sacrifice longevity to a faster reproduction rate.[5]

The scope for change

Extrinsic factors

The first priority in improving the quality of human life is to identify and mitigate deleterious extrinsic factors in lifestyle and environment. There is encouraging epidemiological evidence that this would reduce both the frequency and duration of disability in later life. By delaying the onset of disabling disease to later ages when intrinsic ageing has raised fatality by reducing adaptability, the average duration of disability before death will be shortened. In brief we will spend a longer time living and a shorter time dying. As noted above, this already seems to be happening now in the USA.

Intrinsic ageing

Genetically controlled intrinsic ageing determines maximum lifespan, which is a species characteristic easier to conceptualise than to measure. Given that it is determined by the failure of genes to deal with stochastically distributed damage, maximum lifespan of individuals will show stochastic variation. There is no fixed span and the survival curve of a population is asymptotic to zero. The more data we accumulate the rarer will be the extreme events we are able to observe. The maximum lifespan, as measured by the longest life observed will therefore increase over time even though nothing in biological terms has altered. The numbers but not the proportion of people recorded as surviving beyond 115 will increase with time. For this reason among others, the impact of intrinsic ageing may be more objectively assessed from the rate of rise of age-specific mortality rates than from observed maximum lifespan.

If we wish to attack intrinsic ageing we need to reduce the rate of damage or improve the efficiency of damage control. Experiments are under way aimed at reducing the damage from free oxygen radicals generated by energy production in the mitochondria in cells. Modifying the efficiency of damage control genes is problematic. In the first place we do not know how many of them would need to be identified nor how their action might be made more efficient. The genetic distance between the chimpanzee with a lifespan of 40 years and man with a maximum lifespan around 120 is small, and this may mean that relatively few genes may be responsible. Single genes that materially affect lifespan in lower animals are being discovered and their modes of action elucidated. We should not expect that any of these genes will be found to produce a chemical that would act as an injectable elixir of life to be patented and sold at great profit. Species have evolved to a point of maximum efficiency. All body systems will be tuned to the same length of survival because it would be wasteful of resources and reduce reproduction rate for things to be otherwise. While it might not be strictly necessary to find and modify all the genes affecting damage control, they will function in a network that sets constraints on the overall effects of changing the action of any of its individual components.[6] In a crude analogy, the lifespan of a car will not be lengthened by improving the engine if this increases wear on the transmission or replacement tyres are unavailable.

There may be natural sources of variation that can be manipulated. Some of the genes affecting ageing rates in lower animals work as metabolic switches determining the allocation of resources to reproduction and damage control.[7] In rodents a reversible metabolic switch may underlie the lifespan lengthening effect of caloric restriction.[8] The biological function of this mechanism is to facilitate the survival of individuals during periods of famine. Similar mechanisms may be present in the human. Examples include the amenorrhoea induced by low body weight and, possibly, adaptation of the metabolism of the fetus to the environment in which its mother is living.[9] It may prove possible to manipulate such switches to affect longevity, although there may be effects on quality of life through a biological link with reproduction.

If genetic modifications are required to modify ageing they will need to affect all, or at least most, body systems and organs. This may raise the issue of genetic engineering of the germline rather than somatic therapy. Ethical and legal objections can be anticipated. Every new means of improving the human race or individuals' control over their lives is inevitably met by priesthoods trying to prevent it and lawyers trying to make money out of it. (In a rational and compassionate world would anyone question the right of a woman of 60 having a baby or a widow to conceive a child from the sperm of her dead husband?) In practice if there is a scientific development that some people want and can pay for, ways will be found of achieving it. This may mean cloning in Cambodia and mutations in Mexico. Ideological constraints on scientific development will restrict its benefits to the rich and powerful.

There are therefore good grounds for scepticism about claims that immortality or massive increases in human lifespan are within the general grasp in the next half century. Apart from the complexity of the science involved, prolonging maximum lifespan by modulation of intrinsic ageing processes will require a lifelong approach for greatest effect. Even if we started now therefore we could not expect to see much result within 50 years.

On the other hand, assuming no catastrophes or epidemics of new diseases, we should anticipate a continuation of the present modest steady increase in average lifespan among genetically and socially homogeneous groups in economically developed and politically stable countries. One has to specify "genetically and socially homogenous groups" because racial and social class differences must be expected to remain. Class differences may even widen in the UK. This will be partly because even if there were to be political will to reduce class disparities in education, housing, and lifestyle, significant determinants of longevity lie in infancy and childhood and it will be more than a generation before the effects of past deprivations are "washed out" of the population. Moreover as society becomes more "just" (as a meritocracy perceives justice) the more intelligent, better educated and more readily acculturated move out of the lower classes, leaving only the least endowed behind. This process, essentially one of redefinition of the lower classes, has undoubtedly contributed to the much bewailed widening of social class differences in the UK since the Second World War. Social Darwinists from Huxley down to Thatcher would see this merely as an inevitable manifestation of a successfully competitive society and pass by on the other side. Compassion calls for something rather more from an economic system that serves most of us pretty well but some of us abominably. But we stray beyond our brief.

The progress of medicine

New possibilities for prolonging high quality life in the next half century arise from innovative approaches to the management of diseases and disabilities. Recent decades have seen exciting developments in rational pharmacology based on the identification of cell receptors and an understanding of stereochemistry. Other themes likely to develop include autografting and new approaches to targeting and destroying undesirable cells.

In some conditions, for example Parkinson's disease, there is hope for benefit from replacing dying or degenerate cells in particular situations. At present, experiments are based on the use of fetal cells as being less likely to be rejected by the immune system of the recipient. We can anticipate that transplantation of human cells between different individuals (homografts) will be replaced by cells from the recipient's own tissues. Transplants of non-human tissues (xenografts) are unlikely to provide a long-term option, both for practical reasons and because of the dangers of passage of zoonotic infections.

Replacement of cells might be achieved by a variety of techniques. At the simplest level, chemical messengers such as growth factors may suffice to stimulate cells to regenerate in situ. More complex options will include the manipulation of intra-nuclear mechanisms of epigenetic control to switch specific genes on or off to determine the morphology or function of cells. Using such techniques, undifferentiated cells harvested from a person's bone marrow might be stimulated to grow into heart or brain cells in the laboratory and then grafted back into appropriate situations in the donor's tissues as autografts. There is a recent hint that the capacity of some amphibians to regrow complex tissues and organs such as an amputated limb may be latent in some mammalian species and potentially reproducible in man.

There has been much enthusiasm over the discovery that telomerase can prolong the survival of human cells in culture.[10] The relevance of limitation in lifespan of cultured cells to ageing of the intact organism is not straightforward as few of us die because of exhaustion of reproductive capacity in tissue cell lines. The potential significance of telomerase, and other means of restoring and preserving the reproductive capacity of cell lines, lies in the possibility for replenishing tissues destroyed by disease. Telomerase may provide a means of putting back the clock on cell division preparatory to directing the genetic programme of cells down

177

particular pathways.

The need for specific connections of cells may limit the immediate applicability of autografting. If we could take stem cells and drive them to develop as dopaminergic neurons however, we might have a means of replacing the defective nuclei in Parkinson's disease. There is reason to believe that this could work at least to a limited extent because secretion of dopamine in the relevant nuclei is thought to work in part as a general neuromodulator rather than a cell-to-cell specific messenger. There is an analogous possibility that autotransplantation of cholinergic cells could produce the benefits seen by the use of cholinergic medication in Alzheimer's disease. This affects predominantly the memory deficit subserved by neurons subserving memory in the hippocampus and mamillary bodies. In the later stages of the disease wider problems in cognition, reasoning and speech develop as cortical cells are destroyed by the Alzheimer process. Replacing these cortical cells in an effective way is likely to depend on the connections the transplanted graft can make with other cells. In other words it will be the pattern of wiring not just the ability to secrete particular chemicals that will matter. Perhaps grafted cells will find their own way to appropriate associations but the environment of the mature brain is likely to differ from the developing organ in which such connections are automatic.

Much more promising is the information being gained on the pathogenetic mechanisms of Alzheimer's disease, offering the promise of chemical interventions to arrest the processes poisoning the cells of the brain. Further off, but perhaps awaiting no more than a single crucial insight, is knowledge of the causes rather than just the mechanisms of the disease.

A further theme for medicine of the third millennium will comprise new approaches to targeting, penetrating and destroying or modifying cells. The ability to target specific cells in the body for the delivery of therapeutic agents has long been a dream of medicine. Antibiotics reach all cells but destroy bacteria by interfering with vital chemical processes that are not shared by the body's cells. Some other agents are preferentially taken up by cells with specific chemical functions. Iodine is concentrated in the thyroid gland for example and chemicals concentrated in bone or liver are used for imaging and therapy. Knowledge of surface receptors on specific cells can be exploited to achieve penetration of the cell membrane and targeting of contents including DNA. Knowledge of the genome of antibiotic-resistant bacteria combined with custom-made molecules, perhaps based on viral models, could be used to introduce anti-sense messenger molecules into bacterial cells. This might provide the next phase in the war on antibiotic-resistant bacteria. Analogous approaches to cancer cells may render the crude approaches of surgery and chemotherapy obsolete. These developments will be of benefit to old as well as young.

The organisation of medical care

There are clouds on the horizon for the NHS. The treatments envisaged above, especially those based on autografting, are unlikely to be cheap, nor would it be realistic to expect the costs to be offset by savings on conventional care. The NHS is already creaking at the joints owing to the unacknowledged problem of under-funding. The UK currently spends £800 per person per year on health while the average for the European Community is £1100. The middle classes are making up the difference for themselves with private health insurance, but this is not an option for the poor. Within the next 50 years we can expect the politicians to run out of excuses for the failure of the NHS to keep up with the health services of other nations. If it is to be continued people will have to fund it at a realistic level. This will almost certainly require facing up to the rationing decisions that present governments are ducking. If the NHS is to be destroyed we will sink to the American two-standard model. This would mean more than a change in our health system. The NHS has become the conscience of the nation in its founding commitment to our bearing each others' burdens. Its loss would permanently change the relationship between citizens, and not for the better.

At a professional level, the balance between generalism and specialism will continue to be an issue in medicine. Whatever happens to the trajectory of ageing, multiple pathology will continue to accumulate as the years of life pass. The generalist physician will continue to be needed, but the old model of the generalist with a special interest will become obsolete as those special interests take up more time and training. This will also liberate future generalists to develop a more coherent and rational basis for their work. In a transitional phase, the new generalists would most logically evolve out of the two most broadly relevant of present specialties, geriatrics and clinical pharmacology. Within the last few years younger geriatricians comprise the largest specialty group providing general medical emergency services for adults of all ages in British hospitals. Given contemporary demography, this is entirely logical.

Impact on society

The overall effect of these developments will be to continue the increase in numbers of older people. We must hope that current American experience will be replicated here in that older people will be fitter. Wider futures open before us if, as seems possible, new generations of older people prove to be more politically active than their predecessors. Disillusionment with broken promises and institutionalised corruption of political parties may enhance the essentially democratic process of tactical voting. Solidarity will extend further down the age range because people forcibly retired at 45 or 50 will see common cause more with the older than with their younger fellow citizens. There will be many implications. Using poverty and deprivation of the old to subsidise the affluence and services for the young will no longer be a soft political option. Changes in employment practices will be needed to provide older people with decent pensions. This will necessitate removal of present deterrents to the employment of older people, perhaps including the practice of salaries increasing with age. If these things can be achieved, there will be a general benefit to society as a whole.

Achievement of a significant increase in longevity will probe culturally based ideas of the trajectory of life. The increase in active postretirement life has so far been seen as a flowering of the traditional image of the life trajectory rather than as a challenging innovation. People have always had hopeful visions of Darby and Joan cottages with roses around the door; a Saga Holidays knees-up in Benidorm is merely a modern version of the same old theme of reward for a life of work and subordination to practical need. Will the same image survive postretirement years that outnumber those of work?

Where will the sense of fruition, of the aim and purpose of life be found? Probably not in the family. The charms of great-great-grandchildren may prove uncompelling. Evolutionary biology tells us that our emotional involvement in our progeny will fall off by a factor of 2 for every generation, even without factoring in the cost of birthday presents. There will be personal tragedies in people outliving their inner resources as well as their finances, unless we rethink the whole structure of work, wages, education, and age. All this was pointed out in the Carnegie Report on the Third Age.[11] The resounding silence from government and trade unions with which the Report was greeted is clear indication that nothing will happen until older people use their voting power to coherent purpose.

Contrasted futures

The future is not in our hands. Economically the third millennium will belong to China, but we do not know if it will be the China of Tiananmen Square or whether some new humanist vision may emerge in that unpredictable nation. In Europe the myth of the multicultural society will blow up in our faces through mass migrations of the intolerant and the intolerable. We must dream of a better world, but there is little trust to be put in governments and other rulers of darkness in industry and the media. In the context of clinical futures hope will lie in an alliance between biomedical scientists and the public. This calls for a common language and a common culture between scientists and the citizenry. Yet one cannot but view with sinking heart the present scientific illiteracy of the British public; the chattering classes dwell in a perpetual twilight of the half-baked and ephemeral. Television and weekend colour supplements feed the dwindling attention span of the ill-educated with a titillating pap of half-truth and innuendo. Few members of parliament, or of the administrative class of the civil service, have significant higher scientific education. Perhaps the newly formed Academy of Medical Sciences will see fit to develop a strategic programme of public information.

Envoi

It is in the nature of a geriatrician to be a constructive optimist. That is to say he believes that things can always be made better but are unlikely to become so spontaneously. The third millennium offers plenty of scope for constructive optimism, even though it seems that endless youth is not to be our lot, at least in the foreseeable future. We will continue to grow old, but will take longer over doing it. We will deal more effectively with afflictions along the way. This in itself offers scope for enhancement of human life if we can bring about the necessary adaptations in social organisation. Serial monogamy will no doubt continue to grow in popularity, and older, fitter (and richer) men will have the opportunity to revert to the social habits of our primate ancestors in breeding from a succession of younger consorts.[12] The menopause is no longer a barrier to childbearing for women, although few, one suspects, will wish to repeat indefinitely the dubious joys of child-rearing.

We must re-conceptualise the present trajectory of working into a child-raising period of employment followed by a stage of self-fulfilment, rather than "retirement", which may or may not involve gainful activity. If we can somehow solve the problem of poverty in a postemployment phase of life, exciting opportunities are on offer. The growth of a fitter, more demanding and more politically aware class of older people could catalyse the fundamental changes in post-industrial society that is sorely needed. If the enforced or voluntary leisure of later life can be linked to the opportunities for learning and study provided by the electronic world, older people could become a national resource of knowledge and wisdom. Preretirement courses should focus on the techniques of electronic learning. Discounted subscriptions to the internet may prove more attractive to the next generation of older people than reduced fares on Britain's disintegrating railways. Special interest groups can assemble in cyberspace searching, collating, cataloguing. The potential for abuse however is frightening. The greedy and the intolerant are already closing in on the internet. It may be a freeway in principle but those who can gain control of access to it can insert their own censoring and monitoring filters as an electronic inquisition. Governments fawning on media moguls will not protect us. Nor will those in employment with families to feed want to risk the displeasure of their employers or clients, by standing out for liberty. Far from being a social incubus, the new caste of older people freed from the tangling nets of employment and patronage could be the grey guardians of all our freedoms.

References

1 Hill K, Hurtado M. The evolution of premature reproductive senescence and menopause in human females: an evaluation of the "grandmother hypothesis". *Human Nature* 1991; **2**, 313–50.

2 Williams A. Rationing health care by age. The case for. *Br Med J* 1997; **314**: 8–9.

3 Eliot TS. *Sweeney Agonistes. Collected poems 1909–1932*. London: Faber, 1936.

4 Manton KG, Corder L, Stallard E. Chronic disability trends in elderly United States populations: 1982–1994. *Proc Natl Acad Sci USA* 1997; **94**: 2593–8.

5 Kirkwood TBL, Rose MR. Evolution of senescence: late survival sacrificed for reproduction. *Phil Trans R Soc Lond B* 1991; **332**: 15–24.

6 Kirkwood TBL, Kowald A. Network theory of aging. *Exp Gerontol* 1997; **32**: 395–9.

7 Grimley Evans J. Metabolic switches in ageing. *Age Ageing* 1993; **22**: 79–81.

8 Masoro EJ. Dietary restriction and aging. *J Am Geriatr Soc* 1993; **41**: 994–9.

9 Barker DJP. The fetal origins of diseases in old age. *Eur J Clin Nutr* 1992; **46** (suppl 3): S3–9.

10 Bodnar AG, Ouelette M, Froliks M *et al.* Extension of life-span by introduction of telomerase into normal human cells. *Science* 1998; **279**; 349–52.

11 The Carnegie Inquiry into the Third Age. *Life, work and livelihood in the third age.* Dunfermline: The Carnegie United Kingdom Trust.

12 Harcourt AH, Harvey PH, Larson SG, Short RV. Testis weight, body weight and breeding system in primates. *Nature (Lond)* 1981; **293**: 55–7.

9 Future health scenarios and public policy

Michael Peckham

The clinical "present" benefits from some of the most exciting examples of twentieth century creativity and ingenuity. By contrast, many aspects of the organisation and structure of health care are historical and struggling to contain a revolution in science, technology, and social development. Manifestations of this are the tentative and often ineffectual approaches to chronic illness and preventable disease as well as variations in standards and methods of treating acute problems.

The clinical future can be thought of in two ways: the future of clinical practice and the broader future of which clinical practice forms part. Either way it is clear that the clinical future is necessarily bound up with the future of society. In terms of financing and style it will be influenced by the efforts of governments to balance social development, political freedom, and industrial competitiveness. At present the achievements are un-even. Even in rich countries individuals or even segments of cities are disadvantaged and excluded from many of the health and other benefits enjoyed by the rest of society.

The global economy will increasingly demand a selected range of skills. Education and training criteria will be constantly reviewed to meet those needs and the trend is towards a disconnection between poor and affluent countries. In 1995, for example, only about half of sub-Saharan African countries had access to the internet, the total number of telephone lines was less than those of major cities in the richer countries, and electricity usage per capita was about 20 times less than in the west. This contrasts sharply with trends in affluent countries. For example in 1998 it was reported that the use of the internet in the USA was doubling every 100 days with electronic commerce expanding rapidly and the digital economy accounting for more than 8% of gross domestic product. In 5 years time it is estimated that information technology will account for more than a quarter of USA domestic growth.

As Castells in *The End of the Millennium* has pointed out, one consequence of exclusion is to encourage the emergence of a global economy based on crime. This is already big business, with illegal drugs money exceeding global oil revenues. The implications for health are many. The health of excluded populations and individuals is compromised. Their problems open up threats to others, for example through prostitution and HIV/AIDS, other transmitted diseases, addictive drugs, trading in human spare parts, slavery, child labour, and illicit trading in nuclear material.

These, together with other health consequences of global inequalities, will influence foreign policy driven by self interest as well as by humanitarian considerations. An extended European Union will be well placed to contribute to positive developments in health and medicine through new interfaces with eastern countries, including the former Soviet Union, with Moslem countries through improved relationships with Turkey, and with the South through the North African Mediterranean world. The success of regional groupings between different European states based on economic, cultural and social common interests could lead to new models of international collaboration.

Despite the spectacular advances of medicine and the general improvement in health statistics across the world, the gap between our technological sophistication and social primitiveness is stark. Thus, as mankind prepares to enter the third millennium, it is capable not only of etching nanocircuits with electrons or of performing microsurgery on neonates, but also of engaging in ethnic cleansing and the widespread violation of human rights. This discordance is not new but it is more stark.

Generalism and specialisation

In the communication age, separate "cells" of thinking and action have become more rather than less pronounced. The latter half of the twentieth century has seen a withering of generalism and the emergence of super-specialisation in many fields. In medicine there is fragmentation of what used to be general medicine and general surgery into a growing number of specialties and sub-specialties. The term "general practice" has given way to "primary care" and we can anticipate the demise of the general practitioner as specialisation enters community-based medicine.

Specialisation is not unique to medicine. It brings benefits but it tends to overlook problems particularly those that cut across sectors, disciplines, interests and countries. Because these are the most pressing issues we can anticipate a major emphasis on "holistic" problem solving over the coming decades with an investment in methodologies for connecting and integrating knowledge relating to different fields of activity.

This recalls earlier attempts to bring the range of human knowledge and experience to bear on the problems of governance. Thus when Charles II created the Royal Society in 1662, it was to encourage "the improvement of natural knowledge" by drawing on "all the professions" as well as independent savants – "gentlemen free and unconfined". To this end its membership included not only scientists such as Newton and Boyle, but also architects such as Wren, poets such as Dryden and Cowley, and men of letters such as Pepys and Evelyn.

Over the coming decades the benefits of specialisation will be exploited more successfully within a broad problem-solving context. There will be an emphasis on the transfer of investigative methods and know-how from one field to another. This includes the application to problems in other sectors of experimental methods that have become the norm in medicine. Policy formation has relied on retrospective interpretation and forecasts and on non-systematic ways of acquiring and using evidence. Recently Moses and Mosteller have highlighted studies in education, welfare, justice, medicine and manpower training where prior belief in what was being proposed proved to be misleading. Over half the policy interventions cited did not have a positive effect on the problem they were intended to solve, despite the fact that their proponents believed they were sure winners. They go on to illustrate the power of experimental methods in policy changes relating to speed limits, domestic violence, bail from jail, and educational class size.

The use of experimental techniques will emphasise the limitations of rationality in policy and practice. The conflict between evidence-based decision making and local politics and interests will come to the fore. For example, there may be sound evidence supporting closure of a local children's ward, but this may be resisted for political and other reasons. The tension between rational argument and strongly held but unsupported convictions will become a central issue in health care.

Cities and health

Urban health and the quest for "healthy cities" will attract a high level of interest. During the twentieth century there has been a substantial shift in many countries from agrarian economies to urban living. For example, between 1930 and 1980 the percentage of the population working in agriculture fell from 47% to 11% in Italy, and from 21% to 6% in France. In the early phases of industrial development urban organisation comprised a central business area with a centripetal flow of workers. With changes in the nature of industry and commerce and developments in communications, the monocentric city has given way to "edge cities" and international cities that are nodal points in global networks.

The study of cities began to change in the 1980s, based on new concepts about the way in which local decisions and actions result in patterns that define the nature of the urban environment. As described by Michael Batty, the principle of self-organisation, drawing on chaos theory, simulation, and spatial analysis, is providing a new basis for planning, interventions, and the management of complexity. Even large cities are based on an amalgamation of entities – villages or towns – that vary in character, affluence, employment rates, health status, and safety. Fresh concepts of bottom-up urban evolution will allow the physiology and pathology of city "village" development and the determinants of "health" and "ill health" to be better understood. Teasing out the requirements for urban health and understanding the dynamics of collaboration between different local interest groups will become a key area of investigation.

The dazzling 2040s

Images of what we have seen can be called up and viewed in the "mind's eye" consciously, or involuntarily as in dreams. Not all past images are available to us and a selection is made over which the individual has little control. Some images are partial, others vividly complete, and occasionally there is an unexpected flashback to a long-stored visual memory. Up until 2040 only painters could transfer these mind's eye images into an approximated external form on canvas. Otherwise the vast human visual repository remained secret and locked away. A period of rapid progress in neuro-transmitter science and synaptic drug development, together with major advances in functional imaging, led to a method for tapping into the visual archive and displaying the complete sequence of pictures winding back as necessary to specific events. The significance for forensic science and criminal investigation was obvious. It raised many other issues including the confidentially of stored visual images. Since the method was simple and non-invasive it began to be used to probe past behaviour including issues such as fidelity.

Because it was possible, without too much difficulty, to distinguish between images that had actually been seen and those that had been imagined and fantasised, the method achieved widespread use in psychological testing. For obvious reasons people began to dread it. As is often the case with science, inventions tend to stimulate other developments. In this case a few years after externalised visual display techniques were introduced, a new product was isolated from a deep sea shrimp. This proved an effective blocker to the "minds eye" function and prevented displays from being carried out. Whether or not the drug was taken before legally required testing assumed the status of drug abuse in sport in the 1990s.

At about the same time the technique was perfected for the cultivation of organs in individuals who were artificially supported over a crisis period until it was time to harvest the fully grown replacement organ. Organ growth monitoring centres ran a routine service checking and adjusting growth control medication. In the early days surgery was needed to connect the new organ appropriately, but this became unnecessary as vascular and other connections were pro-grammed into the cultivation schedule and targeted apoptotic agents were used to eliminate redundant structures.

In fact, the 2040s saw a burst of technological innovation. Remote-controlled robotic surgery was performed for the first time between the earth and the moon, and nanotechnology finally delivered the molecular machines necessary to transit through the body, repairing defects, enhancing subnormal function, and seeking out and eliminating early pathological change.

A comparable fantasy would have been the description in 1870 of an invisible ray that passed through the body and revealed its inner structure. Even if the discovery of X-rays had been predicted, their impact on science, medicine and even art could not have been foreseen. After the discovery not only the medical and scientific world were excited. Artists had always sought to see beyond outer surfaces to capture the essence of what they were painting. Cabaret liked the idea of a dancing skeleton, and poets and mystics looked forward to visualising the soul. It could not have been foretold that 50 years on X-rays would play a role in working out the structure of DNA, or that a century later, knowledge in the lineage from the discovery of X-rays and natural radioactivity would be used to elucidate brain function – if not to explore the dynamics of the soul.

Genome

In his poem *Genetic Galaxy*, Les Murray conjures up the idea of a sequestered chart that, if revealed, would show an individual's true antecedents and with it some surprises.

> In many a powerless mind
> lurks this chart, wider than the world
> maybe vast enough to wrap earth in
> which diagrams with merciless truth
> the parentage of everyone, identified
> and linked with their red blood kin
> across all of time and space.

Revelation would lead to "howls of posh, unspoken people", it would reveal "cousinship with kulak shooters", "shock historical non-paternities" and the "stratosphere-tightening gasp at incest seen in full". It would be "glorious to see a hero car-bomber shattered by wrong ancestry".

Genomic and genetic research coupled with informatics is today's equivalent of the discovery of X-rays a century ago and the future consequences are as unforeseeable as were the implications of Roentgen's finding. The DNA revolution has had a fairly protracted gestation since the double helix structure of DNA was described in 1953, but all is now rapidly changing, ushering in a new era for diagnosis, treatment, and disease prevention.

In the 1990s it was shown for the first time in sheep that nuclear material from an adult mature cell fused with the enucleated ovum could form an embryo which after implantation in a surrogate mother could go on to produce a normal lamb. The first successful experiment used cells from the udder of a living ewe, but subsequently a lamb has been produced from fused cells cultured in the laboratory. The technology of nuclear transfer demonstrates that mature cells can be persuaded to revert to an embryonic form. Fetal cells have been implanted with some success into the brain of patients with Parkinson's disease. One possibility is for brain cells from individual patients to be dedifferentiated using nuclear

189

transfer methods and implanted back into the donors. Other anticipated applications of nuclear transfer include the production in pigs of organs that are tolerated as xenotransplants in human recipients, also the preparations of cattle, sheep and pigs with the human genetic material for producing human proteins that can be harvested and used to treat patients.

From genomic research we can anticipate novel molecule and protein therapies, the targeting of existing therapies, and the genetic dissection of diagnostic disease categories. Knowledge of genetic risk will influence personal behaviour including eating habits and other behavioural patterns. Population genetic testing will reveal the anatomy of hidden disease and predisease states necessitating a redefinition of "health needs".

The genomic revolution will be driven by advances in silicon microchip technology and robotics allowing molecules generated by computer to rapidly be tested in multiple simultaneous experiments. The results will aid drug discovery, elucidate the role of genes in health and disease and lead to the development of new diagnostic methods. Home-based kits will become available, for example, allowing self-testing for pregnancy and self-monitoring for drug therapy. These new technologies raise the prospect of home-based blood sampling and automated drug prescription.

Knowledge of the genome of pathogenic micro-organisms will yield new methods of disease prevention. A recent report on complete genome sequence of the tuberculosis bacillus noted that "the combination of genomics and bio-informatics has the potential to generate the information and knowledge that will enable the conception and development of new therapies and interventions needed to treat this airborne disease and to elucidate the unusual biology of its aetiological agent, *Mycobacterium tuberculosis*". Vaccine development based on well-characterised antigens, an understanding of antigenic variation, and knowledge of the molecular basis of virulence will lead to new prophylactic and therapeutic interventions as well as to an epidemiological understanding of the spread of disease based on genetic subtyping.

Population genetic testing, new methods of genetic diagnosis and the subclassification of disease categories on the basis of genotype will be short- to medium-term developments. Novel therapeutics and the routine use of therapies involving the transfer of genes into either somatic cells or germ cells of recipients are likely to be further away.

There are consequences for governments in the large scale and rapid industrial developments in genetics and health. Industry invests massively in genetic and genome R&D, as well as in the information systems needed to handle the outputs. Know-how, data, diagnostic tests, and therapies will encourage the move into health care offering testing, screening, treatment, counselling, and population monitoring. Unchallenged this will result in a huge disparity between the commercial and public sectors in terms of knowledge, expertise and technology with implications for costs and equity. Policies will be needed to ensure that genetic information is available to and used appropriately by the public sector.

The genomic era will also lead to a reappraisal of what constitutes individual identity. DNA fingerprinting already provides a precise method of identification. Genes and external features such as iris pigmentation patterns and facial contours, and the dissection of "normality" in terms of the relationships between genes, behaviour, and personality, will extend concepts of individual identity.

Despite initial misgivings genetically modified plants will greatly improve human health. The world population will double by 2030 to 12 billion inhabitants, placing a greatly expanded demand on food production and distribution. The selective breeding of plants has a long history and seeks to optimise the genetic makeup of existing species. In recent years, genes from other organisms have been introduced with a variety of objectives. These include delay in ripening or rotting and resistance to insects, fungal infection and herbicides used to eliminate weeds. Genetically modified maize, soya, rape, potatoes, and cotton are already in widespread use in the USA and are beginning to impact on other countries. Genetically engineered plants will have a role in producing medicinal products such as taxol which would otherwise be extracted from yew trees. Plants with increased levels of vitamins C and E, and beta carotene, and the isolation of the thousands of currently unidentified compounds in plant biochemistry will provide other potential sources relevant to health. Drought-resistant and salt-resistant plants will have obvious potential benefit to poorer countries and on the health of inadequately nourished people.

The advantages are clear and the apprehensions understandable, including concerns about the double interests of companies such as Monsanto that market both the herbicide-resistant seeds and herbicides. The public is also concerned by fears such as the possibility that antibiotic resistance may be transferred from plants into gut bacteria creating pathogens that are dangerous to man. The onus is on manufacturers to demonstrate safety. However, it is clear that genetically modified foods will become mainstream in agriculture.

Cognitive decline

With more than half the current UK population at risk of developing Alzheimer's disease, and with the often catastrophic consequences for family life and family resources, the problem of cognitive failure will attract a high level of future investment and development.

There will be pressure for presymptomatic screening of middle-aged people and perhaps even younger people as pathology and pathogenesis are better understood. A profusion of new medicines will come on stream, including those that act on amyloid pathways. Genotypic analysis, counselling, presymptomatic diagnosis, preventive interventions, and new therapeutic methods can be anticipated. Genetic mutations in the gene encoding amyloid precursor protein and presenelin gene mutations presage the more complete elucidation of genetic determinants and pathological pathways. There is already clear evidence of differences in drug response in relation to genotype, providing the basis for the selective use of therapy.

There will be a convergence of neurodevelopmental and educational research leading to new knowledge about cognitive impairment, and the development of neurostimulatory interventions including an understanding of the protective effects of sustained intellectual activities on the preservation of cognition.

The age of health informatics

Informatics, communications and telemedicine will radically change the nature of health care and medicine. In the next century the duplication of facilities, functions and staff in hospitals dotted across countries and continents will seem an extraordinary aberration. It is difficult to think of any other sector with multiple sites supported by a common set of services. Teleconsultations, telediagnosis and telecare will be in widespread use within and between countries. After a fairly long gestation the first signs of far-reaching changes are discernible. In Malaysia a start has been made connecting community-based health-care facilities with hospital centres to permit aspects of patient care to be conducted at distance.

Through current telemedicine facilities, centralised reading of radiological and other images, diagnostic opinions, for example on retinal images or pigmented and other skin lesions, advice on injuries, advice on complex case management, and home care monitoring such as electrocardiography are all possible and in use. The combination of computer and communications technologies linked to clinical decisions based on research evidence will become highly developed and a powerful means of pursuing the objectives of quality, cost-effectiveness, and equity.

Telemedicine methods will allow patients to have the expert opinions that they might not have otherwise had. For example, routine tertiary specialist opinions via telemedicine will be used to make the best use of highly skilled expertise in order to enhance quality of care and reduce differences in treatment and outcome.

Patient care will be managed through workstations that provide telemedicine facilities, access to routine information and research databases, as well as to electronic patient records. However, the evolution will be slow if current inertia is not overcome. The exploitation of informatics and telecommunications in health care is a prime example of the need for service developments to be firmly based on well-conceived plans. Intended users need to be involved in design, with their feedback influencing technological improvements and practical application.

Worldwide there is enough experience to demonstrate that telemedicine methods work and solve problems in a novel way. It will not replace the social or medical encounters in health care but add value to them. It will have an obvious role to play in linking underprovided populations in remote geographical areas with centres with the requisite level of expertise. For many highly populated industrialised countries the question will be not whether, but how and over what timescale, telemedicine methods can be integrated into health care as a problem-solving technology. Appropriately developed, distance diagnosis and case management advice will reduce the need for buildings, facilities, and personnel. Diagnostic specialists will be concentrated in fewer locations with information transmitted from community settings by non-medical staff.

The uses of information and communication technologies will contribute to the unification of care. Specialisation in medicine means that the individual becomes a potential stamping ground for a large number of disciplines and subdisciplines. The individual may feel that no one is looking at them as a whole and multiple opinions arranged in the conventional way are usually cumbersome and protracted. Telemedicine will provide a mechanism for linking different specialised interests with each other and with general care in the community.

The new technologies will lead to informed consumerism. Television with computing capacity and speech recognition will permit the viewer to determine the use of words, sounds and images with inflow of information as well as outward communication. The technology exists. Its potential for education, training, advice, retailing and linkage between government and people need to be worked out.

The implications for the clinical future are clear. Information in an easily accessed and comprehensible format will allow users to become informed about what is known, the limitations of knowledge, and what can be done to maintain health, to prevent ill health, and to treat disease. A major obstacle might be competing information of uncertain quality made available on the internet by pressure groups. Combined information and computer facilities open the way to home-based diagnosis, advice, health monitoring, and clinical management, particularly of chronic illness. Home access to personal health data as well as to information on professional and institutional characteristics and performance will emerge from the use of this technology.

Within the health-care system, current teething problems with electronic patient records will be overcome and issues of confidentiality resolved. In particular the criteria and *raison d'être* for confidentiality arrangements will be revised to ensure that real needs are being met and dogma not allowed to override common-sense. This is particularly true where confidentiality inhibits the collection and use of information that would be likely to benefit the very individuals who are the intended subjects of protection.

The availability in electronic form of diagnostic, treatment and outcomes information will constitute a huge database which, used appropriately, will make inter- and intra-institutional variations in standards of care and costs of care a historical phenomenon. Such information will provide a routine way of monitoring the results of clinical care and yield valuable insights into natural history, also providing the basis for linking genotypic and phenotypic information.

194

The individual in an interconnected society

In the interconnected society the individual is subsumed into a global milieu. However other trends will give emphasis to individuality. Genetic "uniqueness" will acquire a new dimension as it becomes possible to describe the genes along an individual's genome. Individualisation of therapies will become a reality and genetic contributions to development and behaviour will be elucidated with educational interventions and childrearing tailored to the individual. The use of molecular genetic methods in archaeology and anthropology will transform our knowledge of population movements and cultural origins and challenge preconceived notions of ethnicity and origin.

At the same time, and in response to a technology-dominated world, people will seek "whole person" forms of health care. Already more than 5 million people in the UK each year seek complementary and alternative medicine and doubtless more would if they could afford it. Similar trends are seen in other countries and many of those who go to non-orthodox practitioners are young without known physical symptoms or disability. This quest for holistic care to complement orthodox medicine may reflect the attraction of a one-to-one relationship between patient and the practitioner which used to be a feature of orthodox health care but which is being compromised by rapid throughput, larger primary care groups, and other trends.

Defining the health "problematique"

For any given society, defining what constitutes the set of problems under the label "health" should be a prerequisite for developing and applying appropriate correctives. Currently health problems are articulated from viewpoints that are either too narrowly focused or impossibly diffuse. Over the next two decades there will be a shift away from the economic objectives that have dominated the twentieth century. Health will become a central concern of governments based on a concept of health that emphasises individual creativity. Purposeful living, protection from physical and mental injury and prevention and treatment of disease and disability will be integrated and form the basis for policy decisions.

At present the right words are used but the direction is confused. The Institute of Medicine's "2020 vision", for example, notes that "the positive picture of progress, . . . is counterbalanced by concerns about health inequity and health diversity between and within countries." Contemporary and future issues are identified: environmental threats (air, water, global warming, chemical, ozone depletion), infections (HIV/AIDS, ebola virus, plague, tuberculosis, dengue, cholera), and socio-behavioural pathologies (violence, drug abuse, mental and social illness). In the same report, a global transition is identified from a high mortality, high fertility society to one characterised by low mortality and low fertility and it is suggested that this is likely to continue until about 2050. However, in her concluding remarks, Health Secretary Donna Shalala took a much more focused and parochial view, identifying "six impossible things that must become possible". These were to ensure that the culture of research thrives; to protect academic medical centres and clinical research; to ensure that bioethics are as sophisticated as science; to take a long view of science; to balance the budget; to ensure that citizens understand science. She was, of course, addressing a particular constituency from one vantage point but the lack of a broad multisector perspective was striking.

Another kind of restricted look at the problems is apparent in the 1998 Forward Look of the World Health Organisation, "Life in the 21st century – a vision for all". This suggested that "as the new millennium approaches, the global population has never had a healthier outlook". It went on to say that ". . . the most important pattern of progress now emerging is an unmistakable trend towards a healthier longer life". The report thus offered an encouraging prospect of health from a WHO perspective. It is true that there are grounds for optimism but only provided that ways can be found of tackling problems in the round. The WHO viewpoint is based on average health statistics, and averages unfortunately conceal problems. Civil unrest, wars and other miseries that form part of the daily media round are blips on the march towards the WHO vision of a healthier longer life. Indeed, war, crime and drugs do not figure much in the report.

Health through education

The contrast between the exciting potential that exists for human development and innovation and the reality of social and organisational unpreparedness will lead to a radical reappraisal of educational purposes and methods. The shift away from a job for life in a single organisation to periods of employment in a range of settings demands a new type of educational preparation providing analytical and generic skills that can be applied to a range of problems. The new educational formation will need to ensure sufficient confidence and ability to acquire new knowledge and to relinquish know-how relating to previous activities. This is particularly the case in medicine and health care, where changes provoked by new knowledge, products and processes occur in rapid succession. The connection between education and health will become more clearly demonstrated at all levels. Thus, the educational status of parents is germane not only to their own health but to that of their children, and hence the next generation of adults. The situation for women in particular has deteriorated in some parts of the world with the rise of fundamentalism and the transition from communist and dictator rule to democracy. As social globalisation extends the coming decades will take seriously the anticipated knock on effect of educational insufficiency on children and the influence that this has on their ability to function as responsible and contributory citizens. Investments in the education of children will be associated with the provision of education for their parents where this is needed.

The way in which educational interventions from the early childhood years onwards can positively influence brain development and subsequent behaviour and performance will be the subject of intense investigation and lead to new individualised approaches. The role of education in permitting people to participate in the information revolution is already obvious, as are the potential advantages. These include access to knowledge, employability and active participation in the mainstream of society.

Educational research will draw on health research models such as randomised trials, systematic reviews, and audit of outcomes. As a result, educational interventions will be based on better evidence than is currently the case and the "products" of the educational system will be clarified and measured. The impact of education on a broadly drawn notion of "health" will become a key consideration in national and international policy.

Although the economic needs for a well-educated and well-trained workforce will remain, quality of life and health will also come to the fore as major objectives. Cultural diversity rather than cultural separateness will be pursued through a revised state educational system linked to parental education. This will be seen

197

to offer a more distinctive and superior education than the private sector.

Coherent problem solving and research

Universities and research funding bodies have passed through a turbulent period over the past one or two decades. However the future is likely to see even more change. The quest by governments for a balance between national and global interests and between social, economic and political stability will be reflected in the future expectations of academia. In recent years the conventional role of knowledge creation and education have been supplemented by a contribution to wealth creation and national competitiveness. To this will be added the need to contribute to the solutions of complex policy problems.

Currently research councils and other research funding bodies tend to parcel up problem territories and areas of interest and it is often difficult to obtain funding for cross-cutting issues. If, as seems likely, current arrangements based on five research councils prove inhibitory to research on issues that straddle their spheres of interests, and the interests of government, there will be pressure for a single body to allocate public funds. There will also be pressure for a renegotiated relationship between government and the charitable sector designed to align the research they support with national priorities and to complement more overtly the coverage of publicly funded research.

This will raise wider issues about the role of the voluntary sector which will pick up functions that were previously supported through public funds and develop a more strategic position. Already about half the adult population in Britain is involved in formal voluntary work and this will increase. The National Lottery and new charitable foundations are extending the scope of voluntary sector interventions in the provision of services, health research, and advocacy. The voluntary sector will design, support and test new clinical and health-care models which will then become the responsibility of the public and/or private sectors.

New criteria for the allocation of government funds to the universities will be introduced to encourage interinstitutional networks and cross-cutting problem solving. The new criteria will also ensure that research at the interface with the clinical arena draws on appropriate expertise in social, population and clinical sciences, linking biological and physical research in the broader university setting with efficient ways of translating discoveries into early clinical development.

Widespread concern about imperfections in the arrangements for assessing research applications will peak following public exposure of biased decisions protected by anonymity. Closed, mutually supportive networks operating in major funding bodies will be censored and new arrangements introduced to replace the current peer review system. The revised mechanisms will be designed to prevent domination by prevailing scientific fashion and require that decisions are made explicit and fully justified. The new arrangements will address concerns that the review process perpetuates research in fields that are of interest to applicants and reviewers but that are of little importance nationally or scientifically. The new assessment and allocation criteria will address the currently unresolved problem of balancing the effort between fundamental research and research which is directed to the solution of specific problems. Expert opinion will be supplemented by a broad pragmatic overview of review outcomes to advise on whether investments make sense given other demands on resources.

Health services as obstacles to health

Health services in the form in which we know them today will evolve into new structures in the first decades of the twenty-first century. The change will be driven by the need to deliver a pan-governmental multisector commitment to health development as well as the treatment of disease and disability.

In the case of the British National Health Service, its political profile, media worthiness and public standing tend to place it beyond open debate. However, to disregard the possibility that the health service as presently constructed may become an obstacle to health development will be seen to run counter to the spirit of enlightened thinking that led to its creation in the first place.

A number of trends will allow future change to be presented and accepted as a positive and innovative development. The concept of a national service will be increasingly difficult to sustain with devolution and regionalisation in the UK and common health interests coming to the fore in an enlarged European Union. It will prove frustratingly difficult to tackle many of the broader health and social problems though a service that needs to maintain a capacity for providing high quality specialised medical care. By attempting to face in two directions at once, towards public health as well as towards high technology health care, the NHS will be seen to underexploit technology driven medicine while failing to make a significant impact on societal health problems. Excessive expectations will lead to a growing disillusionment with orthodox medicine as reflected by popular demand for complementary and alternative forms of health care. The result of these trends will be a waning of public support for the NHS in its current form which will be seen as overloaded and unable to fulfil its commitments.

A further disturbing trend will be the apportionment of blame to lower socioeconomic and other disadvantaged groups for their ill health. This will be ascribed to self-inflicted damage through adverse behaviour, poor eating habits and other factors that are judged to be within the power of individuals to change. There will be a discernible shift of opinion favouring safety-net health-care provision for poorer people with the more affluent covered by insurance or self payment. Such arguments will be countered by a better understanding of the NHS contribution to the social fabric as well as to health. The emergence of two-tier health care and the threat to social cohesion will be an added stimulus to the creation of an alternative system.

At the time of the change a retrospective analysis of health and social problems will illustrate the mismatch between what the NHS provided and the real-life problems it sought to address. Of particular concern will be the growing inadequacy of provision for isolated, frail elderly people and the limited success in identifying and dealing with potentially preventable health problems.

The new system will include a well-researched and tested incentives framework for attainable disease prevention and the maintenance of health. Research funds will be invested in the elucidation of relationships between social structures and health. The antenatal and early childhood determinants of adult health will become a central issue in public health and health care.

The evolution outlined above will reflect the fact that, despite policy changes and reforms, old health service structures that are ill adapted to change will be seen to linger on: the distinctive architecture and ambience of the "historical" hospital; old fashioned communications systems; inertia in documenting the products of health care.

In future it will be unthinkable not to apply the best that can be achieved with current knowledge, skills and resources with a reasonable level of uniformity in health care. Professional leaders and their constituencies will refocus UK health care on outcomes rather than on content. If this task is neglected and if the gap between the effort devoted to research and technological development on the one hand and practical application to produce measurable health benefits on the other is not closed, it will increase regulation, weaken professional commitment, and cast doubts about the value of research.

Health systems will be obliged to demonstrate that they meet the needs of their users. Looking back it will seem an extraordinary aberration that variations in standards of care were allowed to persist in a technologically sophisticated era dominated in other sectors by consumer choice. In the twenty-first century, we will be astounded at the permissiveness of late twentieth century health care with wide variation in hospital referral rates and the rates at which different procedures are performed; for example, the fourfold difference in the rates of performing coronary artery revascularisation procedures between different health authorities, with the highest rates in those areas with the least need.

At present it is uncertain whether the concept of the "customer" is relevant to the NHS and if so who the customers are: the government which pays for the service from general taxation; or the consumer as a co-payer and taxpayer; or local payers – health authorities and primary care groups. Criteria and mechanisms for establishing consumer needs will be introduced together with clearly defined and workable accountability arrangements to the public and to government. In addressing customer needs it will be necessary to clarify what kind of intervention is most appropriate to meet those needs. This may be a social rather than a health intervention. "Total problem" strategies will be devised to avoid problems, such as obesity, becoming medicalised. As John Vaisey observed, ". . . ill health could be defined as what the doctor decides: it is created or accepted in a medical consultation, thereafter the medical machinery starts up and whatever the problem a medical solution is looked for". Since the potential for increasing technological complexity is practically unlimited, judging the right level of technical sophistication in health care will be crucially important. In the absence of any agreed criteria the pursuit of quality could also be taken to extreme lengths with concomitant demands on resources.

Development and innovation: a new departure

"Health" is the object of or the pretext for a vast national and international research and development effort in both industry and universities. The fruits of this huge investment are knowledge, trained personnel, new products, and new ways of doing things. Information derived from industrial and academic R&D together with the results of evaluations of effectiveness and cost-effectiveness provides the raw material for the development of health care.

Innovation, through finding new ways of using old techniques or through the invention of new technologies, changes the way medicine is practised and this in turn feeds back into the type of facilities needed, the manpower required, the flow of patients, and other modifications to existing services. At the origin of policies formed centrally are changes that have already started to happen at grass roots level. A good example is the development of endoscopy, leading to minimally invasive surgery, the emergence of day surgery, and new hospital requirements.

Despite the fact that health care, perhaps more than any other sector, is presented with a profusion and great diversity of new methods and is subject to constant change, development and innovation are concepts and functions that have had a remarkably low profile in the NHS. Yet the affordable exploitation of new opportunities should have the highest priority. Currently the NHS as an organisation is slow to respond to new challenges. Innovation is often seen as a threat. It is difficult to know how to gain entry to the system in order to interest senior decision-makers in potentially valuable new developments. A good current example is telemedicine.

The coming decades will see the concept of growth and productivity introduced into health care drawing on and adapting industrial models to the specific purposes of a public service. "Growth" in health care will be thought of in two ways. First, the extent to which public health and health services are able to accommodate and absorb the increasing number of new technologies. Second, the extent to which these are deployed in an expanding pool of "consumers", for example, elderly people or those who have intractable conditions for whom treatment will become available. Statements of productivity will be based on what is achieved with constrained resources in terms of cures, preventive interventions, changes in health status and quality of life, new developments and exploited intellectual property.

The notion of competitiveness also has relevance to the health service but in a different context to that of industry. Publicly funded health care competes with other government departments for resources as well as the demands of other sectors for public funds. Health services contribute to national competitiveness through the health of the workforce and the population, through social advancement; through efficient and effective handling of resources, and through exportable innovation.

At present there is no well-defined mechanism for incorporating new technologies and processes in a systematic way to further the development of health-care provision. New medical and other interventions together with the analyses of clinical trials and systemic reviews form, as it were, a predevelopmental depository without there being any clearly cut procedures for drawing upon and exploiting the contents. In particular there is no dedicated development and innovation capacity underpinning the design and implementation of policies that make use of new opportunities to address the priorities of government.

To address these deficiencies a "Technology Gateway" will be introduced into health care. Its functions will be based on preset criteria and serve to screen entry into the health-care system of new forms of practice and to provide an exit mechanism for those that have been superseded or found to be unnecessary or ineffective. The technology gateway will be the means by which the relationship between R&D, policy formation and health care will be formalised. The criteria by which decisions are reached will be drawn up with input from the range of interests involved in health care, including contributions from professional and lay people. They will be based on economic measures and health outcomes – including changes in health status as perceived by patients – and take into account other factors such as emergent developments and the envisaged level of technological complexity to be sustained by the NHS.

Although it is evident that development and innovation are essential ingredients of policy formation, in future this will be made explicit and given high priority with the necessary skills brought to bear from inception though design to implementation. The NHS R&D function must play a key role, extending its remit beyond evaluation to information synthesis and the design of policy, focusing on development and innovation both in relation to policy and practice.

A new development and innovation framework designed to close the gap between the availability of research-based and routine information on the one hand and patient care on the other will form the basis for clinical, professional and heath-care development. Academic hospitals and their associated medical schools have had few incentives to tackle this deficiency. The Higher Education Funding Council's national research assessment exercise has skewed medical school research away from what might be termed translational or impact science. Thus cell and molecular science tends to be juxtaposed physically and organisationally to the clinical interface, with epidemiology, social sciences, economics, evaluation and other ingredients of a balanced health research portfolio often placed in a subsidiary position. While research into biological mechanisms is crucial to provide the breakthroughs needed for new treatments and methods of preventing disease, the organisation of medical schools in relation to the wider arena of university and industrial research needs to be restructured.

Academic medical centres will take the lead in setting in place a capacity for development and innovation with clinical units, ensuring that at least one member of staff is given the remit of concentrating on developmental issues, combining this function with clinical practice. Hospital-based development and innovation staff will be co-ordinated by the institution's director of R&D with a remit to link with and contribute to the health-care knowledge base, to have input to policy development and implementation, to introduce and apply measures of outcome, to further links with industry, and to foster the translation of laboratory and other discoveries into clinical practice. These institutional groupings will extend to district hospitals and primary care and collectively form a national network. This will be drawn upon centrally by policy formers and be called upon to spearhead the implementation of policy. Incentives to move along this route will be strengthened by including in the criteria for allocating R&D infrastructural funds a requirement to demonstrate the presence of effective mechanisms for implementing research findings and for documenting the results of treatment.

Revising the internal milieu of medical schools and teaching hospitals will lead to new strategies for establishing external linkages with primary and community care and social services. Viewed from the twenty-first century contemporary hospitals will seem remarkably like moated castles, slow to exert influence to identify and take steps to correct anomalies outside their intramural interests. It will be a cause of amazement that although women with mammographically detected breast cancer in the South East of England were treated in a variety of different ways that almost certainly compromised survival, this was not apparently a cause of concern to specialised breast cancer units in the same region.

The future of medicine

The goals of medicine have been the subject of reports in the UK and USA and other countries. They follow a similar pattern – they are all embracing, rather general, and not all that helpful.

Medicine is in a quandary. Is its prime function to care for the sick? Is it to prevent ill health? Or should it do both? Where does "medical" responsibility for caring for the sick begin and end? Prevention of sickness extends from medical interventions such as vaccination through to ways of tackling social and economic causes of ill health, and wider global influences such as environmental damage. Where in this spectrum is the physician to play a part? At present the answers to these questions are not clear cut and there is a degree of polarisation between the "biomedical" doctor and the "public health" doctor, as there is between medical and non-medical professionals.

Overall the public continues to hold doctors in high esteem. If difficult resource decisions and choices have to be made the public overwhelmingly feels that these should be made by doctors and not governments or managers. However, this could change. The medical profession needs urgently to contribute to a clarification of its future role because far-reaching decisions will be taken over the next few decades. There are a number of pointers to future change. The first is the trend towards complementary and alternative methods of health care. Another is for nurses to assume greater responsibility for patient care. Other professional staff such as pharmacists are also extending their remit, managers have become firmly established in health care and many would argue that the public health function could be discharged perfectly well by non-medical personnel. At the same time, the trend in medicine is towards increasing specialisation with the creation of larger groups of primary care physicians. Both trends risk distancing patients from doctors in terms of total care. Also lay people are becoming more informed, making use of their access to information including the internet and coming to consultations better armed with knowledge.

These trends could point to a largely technical role for doctors confined to the "high tech" end of health care with other functions performed by non-medical staff. Patient contacts would be predominantly with non-medical personnel with tele-linkages to the specialist. The doctor would then become as remote from his patients as the airline pilot is from his passengers.

If this scenario is to be substantially different, education, training and attitudes must be transformed. Medicine has fought a defensive position over health reforms and many other matters. Today it is not clear where the thinking presence of medicine resides or whether any of the colleges and associations are free enough from their historical interests to examine "clinical futures" with sufficient detachment.

The "new medicine" will be created in an undergraduate environment that is as free as possible from the burden of historical legacies. The medical course will be infused with fresh approaches to provide an enlightened and enlightening education with the range of social sciences integrated with biological and physical sciences and an emphasis on problem analysis and on the uses of knowledge. Students will have exposure to other ways of looking at problems in a range of community, academic and industrial settings. During the educational years the analysis of problems will be seen as more important than research. Throughout there will be contact with patients, their families, and former patients. Students will have access to "mentors" drawn from within or outside academia and from the visual arts, music, theatre, literature or other fields providing an insight into ways of looking at human problems and of working that are distinct from medicine and health care.

Research funding bodies will invest in innovative approaches to medical education basing their support on quality of design, testing, and evaluation. Students will be invited to rate their teaching and institutions would follow the careers of their alumni and make known student outcomes in bids for infrastructural funding.

In contrast with needs, current thinking is limited. Recent proposals for courses on literature and humanities in the existing medical curriculum do not reflect a serious attempt to get to grips with the problems and the remedy prescribed is as arbitrary as Shaw's pound of greengages.

In concept and design, the new medical education will have relevance to a socially and technologically complex environment.

The scope for flexibility and change within existing institutions is probably too limited to foster creative solutions and a new medical school in a broadly based university campus would offer the chance of pioneering the new methods that are urgently needed.

Beyond the educational period the performance of senior doctors as advisors, teachers and mentors will be assessed with external non-medical input. Junior staff will be invited to add their own assessments. In turn junior staff will be assessed not only for their professional performance but the quality of their relationships with patients and other staff.

Third millennium physicians will be surprised that their predecessors were apparently inured to the high levels of stress and anxiety in young doctors. They might note the high level of use of a stress counselling service set up in 1996 for doctors, medical students and their families. Also the fact that a high number of calls related to bullying and intimidation, with older doctors the main cause of the problem. As a counselling services manager commented at the time "treating juniors as the lowest form of life, insensitivity towards colleagues and lack of concern for their well-being are all expected and part of the institution".

A few anecdotes might survive the passage of time, showing how fear of impaired career prospects inhibited junior doctors from seeking help. A medical dean, two or three decades hence, might suffer an unfortunate fate if he followed the example of his 1990s forerunner who advised a young woman doctor, worried about her career, that it was time "she went away and had babies". He might not know that she felt she could not discuss her problem for fear of spoiling her chances of getting a job or that some undergraduates of the day described their student experience as "education by humiliation".

Today, the closed nature of health institutions is illustrated by the twofold variation between different hospitals in the percentage of personnel that are stressed. There are microcultures with different atmospheres, different ways of doing things and differences in facilities even though each institution forms part of one system and has comparable responsibilities. Those who exhibit the highest stress levels are those who are not part of a clinical team. Conversely those who are members of a clinical team are the least stressed. The UK method of organising hospital-based medical staff into consultant firms encourages isolation both of medical decision making and of support when something goes wrong. This structure will be reappraised in relation to other models such as the

Chef de Service approach in other European countries.

Two generations on, the physicians of the day will also reflect on their forebears' lack of emphasis on or interest in the products of health care. They will note that quality judged in terms not only of accuracy of diagnosis and content of care but also of results was virtually non-existent in the late twentieth century NHS, despite a large investment of funds, a mountainous literature and a plethora of conferences and strategic statements on audit and outcomes. In many services clinical audit will be seen to have been an alibi for not getting to grips with measuring the results of health care. The lack of a serious attempt to come to terms with this fundamental aspect of medicine will be seen to have had serious consequences, as illustrated by the case in 1998 of the paediatric cardiac surgeons in Bristol. Here unacceptably high mortality rates were allowed to go unchallenged by those in command despite a protest by others in the same institution. As there was no requirement to make known expected results to patients and their families, they were left in ignorance. The tragic Bristol experience led to a radical change of attitude by and towards the medical profession. The documentation of clinical outcomes became a routine part of patient care with new mechanisms introduced to ensure professional regulation.

The historically minded third millennium clinician will look back and reflect on the time it took for medicine and health care to focus on results. They will reflect on the fate of early pioneers of "outcomes" such as Semmelweiss in the mid nineteenth century who lost his job for introducing hand-washing to combat puerperal sepsis and Codman, who likewise lost his job, in the early twentieth century, for audaciously suggesting to his surgical colleagues in Boston that they should document the results of their operations.

Conclusion

Franz Vranitsky, a former Austrian Chancellor, is said to have commented that "anyone with visions needs to see a doctor". It is true he was referring to Europe rather than health. However if the past is anything to go by attempts to predict future changes in medicine are generally wildly inaccurate.

Nevertheless looking at the future may have some merits. It may alert us to opportunities which would otherwise be downplayed or missed, or prevent us taking steps that inadvertently block fruitful lines of action or enquiry. A view of the future may help shape society and prepare individuals to live with and master new technologies. Finally, by detaching ourselves, if only transiently, from daily routine in order to reflect on what might come, we may be able to see contemporary problems and potential solutions more clearly.

Conversely, forecasting could delude us into making unwise decisions, to have unreasonable expectations or it might even provide alibis for inaction; on balance however the benefits outweigh the disadvantages.

Rather than a futuristic exploration, the emphasis here has been on problems that need to be solved and some of the opportunities for change. In particular the future must see an integration of scientific medicine within a broader framework that tackles social and other determinants of health. This is not an "either or" choice but an absolute requirement if there is to be a balanced approach to health development.

Index

cardiovascular 128–31, 151–2
in childhood 151–2
detection 37–9
genetic prediction 35–6
robotics, medical 59–62, 71, 188
benefits 61–2
in cancer surgery 80–1
definition 59
future developments 60–1
in radiotherapy 58
Royal Society 186
rubella 153

schistosomiasis 77
schizophrenia 96, 97, 100–1, 109
school health service 163–4
scientific education 121–2, 181
screening 21, 35
cancer 21, 35, 78
genetic 8–9, 154–5, 167
preconceptual 154–5
risk factor 38
selection
embryo 80, 101, 135
iatric 9
natural 23–4
self-help approaches 91–2
self-organisation 187
senile plaques 114
sensing 52–6, 69–70
in vitro 53–4
in vivo 54–5, 70
sensitive periods, brain
development 164–5
sexual intercourse, age at first 152
sildenafil 16
single gene disorders 24–5, 37
single nucleotide polymorphisms
(SNP) 33–5
single photon emission
tomography (SPECT) 56
skin, artificial 67
"smart home" technologies 49
smoking 76, 97, 114, 149
social deprivation 7, 135, 180
society
assistive technologies and 48
future 184
interconnected 195
population ageing and 180–1

socioeconomic status
ageing and 176
child health and 150–1
health and 7, 200
socio-nursing professionals 14
specialisation, medical 13, 14,
185–7, 205
speech synthesisers 50
spinal cord injuries 69, 106
SQUID devices 69
statins 123, 142
stem cell transplantation 104–5,
136–7, 177–8
stents, vascular 124, 138
stress 106–8
in doctors 207–8
stroke 96, 98, 128
risk factors 129–30
treatments 111–13
substance abuse 97, 101, 114–15
substance P 110
suicide vectors 86–7
surgery
cancer 80–1
cardiovascular 63–4, 65–6, 141
computer assisted (CAS) 59–60,
61–2
fetal 157
paediatric 160–1
robotics 59–62

teams, clinical 207–8
technology
in cardiovascular medicine
123–4, 138–9
new 202–5
styles of development 18
Technology Gateway 203
telemanipulators, master/slave
61–2
telemedicine 57, 139, 192–4
telesurgery 62, 81, 160
telomerase 177–8
termination of pregnancy 155, 157
thalidomide disaster 2–3
T helper cells, tumour response 85
thought, habits of 2–4
"thrifty genotype" 27, 130–1
thrombolytic drugs ("clot
busters") 112, 123